AF566463

Perspiration Research

Current Problems in Dermatology

Vol. 51

Perspiration Research

Volume Editors

Hiroo Yokozeki Tokyo
Hiroyuki Murota Osaka
Ichiro Katayama Osaka

61 figures, 41 in color, and 10 tables, 2016

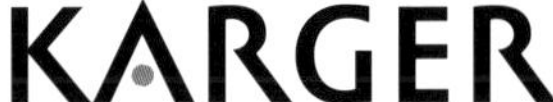

Basel · Freiburg · Paris · London · New York · Chennai · New Delhi · Bangkok · Beijing · Shanghai · Tokyo · Kuala Lumpur · Singapore · Sydney

Current Problems in Dermatology

Hiroo Yokozeki
Department of Dermatology
Graduate School of Medical and Dental Sciences
Tokyo Medical and Dental University
1-5-45 Yushima, Bunkyo-ku
Tokyo 113-8519 (Japan)

Hiroyuki Murota
Department of Dermatology
Course of Integrated Medicine
Graduate School of Medicine
Osaka University
2-2 Yamadaoka, Suita-shi
Osaka 565-0871 (Japan)

Ichiro Katayama
Department of Dermatology
Course of Integrated Medicine
Graduate School of Medicine
Osaka University
2-2 Yamadaoka, Suita-shi
Osaka 565-0871 (Japan)

Library of Congress Cataloging-in-Publication Data

Names: Yokozeki, Hiroo, editor. | Murota, Hiroyuki, editor. | Katayama, Ichiro, editor.
Title: Perspiration research / volume editors, Hiroo Yokozeki, Hiroyuki Murota, Ichiro Katayama.
Other titles: Current problems in dermatology ; 51. 1421-5721
Description: Basel ; New York : Karger, [2016] | Series: Current problems in dermatology, ISSN 1421-5721 ; vol. 51 | Includes bibliographical references and index.
Identifiers: LCCN 2016030383| ISBN 9783318059045 (hard cover : alk. paper) | ISBN 9783318059052 (eISBN)
Subjects: | MESH: Sweating--physiology | Sweat Gland Diseases
Classification: LCC RL141 | NLM WR 102 | DDC 616.5/60072--dc23 LC record available at https://lccn.loc.gov/2016030383

Bibliographic Indices. This publication is listed in bibliographic services, including Current Contents® and Index Medicus.

www.karger.com
Printed on acid-free and non-aging paper (ISO 9706)
ISSN 1421–5721
e-ISSN 1662–2944
ISBN 978–3–318–05904–5
e-ISBN 978–3–318–05905–2

Contents

Online supplementary material: www.karger.com/book/toc/271839

Preface

Many investigators worldwide, particularly those in Japan, have performed leading studies on perspiration. In this book, I provide a history of studies on the physiology of perspiration and other research on perspiration. Particularly, I introduce in detail two historical physiologists: Dr. Yasu Kuno, a former professor at Nagoya University who dramatically revealed the physiology of perspiration in the early and maturation stages, and Dr. Kenzo Sato, a former professor at the University of Iowa. These Japanese investigators have played major roles in perspiration research.

Perspiration research developed dramatically in the 2000s. It has since been elucidated that perspiration not only has a temperature-regulating function and a non-slip function for the hands and feet, but also a natural bactericidal function through dermcidin, an antimicrobial peptide contained in sweat. Moreover, we propose that obstruction of the sweat glands plays a major role in the onset of disorders such as parapsoriasis, lichen planus, and lichen amyloidosis, and that *Malassezia* is an allergen in sweat that exacerbates atopic dermatitis and cholinergic urticaria, making perspiration abnormalities possible causes of many allergic skin disorders. Furthermore, sweat glands were found to play numerous roles, including as storage of stem cells for replenishing epidermal cells in the case of thermal burns and as water retention sites for replenishing moisture in the stratum corneum. We also introduce an analysis of the 3-dimensional structures of the sweat glands in disorders such as dyshidrosis by using high-speed en-face optical coherence tomography (OCT), which can visualize the sweat glands dynamically and 3-dimensionally. OCT provides 3-dimensional imaging by using optical interference; it visualizes the structures of biological tissues under the epidermis at a high resolution and can display the structure of the sweat ducts in the stratum corneum and the epidermis. Furthermore, we demonstrate that sweat and the sweat glands can be visualized by using 2-photon excitation fluorescence microscopy in mice. These 3-dimensional analyses of the sweat glands are likely to unravel novel pathologies of skin disorders in the near future. I hope everyone who reads this book will develop more interest in investigations on perspiration.

Hiroo Yokozeki, Tokyo
Hiroyuki Murota, Osaka
Ichiro Katayama, Osaka

Yokozeki H, Murota H, Katayama I (eds): Perspiration Research.
Curr Probl Dermatol. Basel, Karger, 2016, vol 51, pp 1–6 (DOI: 10.1159/000446750)

New Pathologies of Skin Disorders Identified from the History of Perspiration Research

Hiroo Yokozeki

Department of Dermatology, Graduate School of Medical and Dental Sciences, Tokyo Medical and Dental University, Tokyo, Japan

Abstract

This chapter introduces the history of perspiration research and the latest perspiration research findings. Many investigators worldwide, particularly those in Japan, have carried forward globally leading studies on perspiration. This chapter will introduce the history of studies on the physiology of perspiration and perspiration research by classifying it in three stages, namely the early, maturation, and development stages, with a focus on Japanese researchers who have played active roles in each stage. In particular, I will introduce two historical physiologists in detail, Dr. Yasu Kuno, a former professor of Nagoya University, who dramatically revealed the physiology of perspiration in the early and maturation stages, and Dr. Kenzo Sato, a former professor of the University of Iowa.

Early Stage of Perspiration Research

In 1775, Blagden published the first paper on perspiration research, showing that humans perspire to cool body temperature whereas dogs cool their bodies by panting when it is hot without perspiring, which he discovered by taking a sauna bath with a dog while measuring its body temperature [1]. In 1833, Purkinje discovered the sweat gland, and his pupil Wendt published a research paper on this finding [1]. Through the 1930s, the following basic items were already established in the physiology of perspiration: (1) humans and other animals have different mechanisms to control perspiration, (2) humans have eccrine and apocrine glands that have different anatomical structures and distributions, (3) perspiration from the eccrine glands is induced by heat, mental excitement, and taste stimulation, and (4) perspiration from the eccrine glands is innervated by sympathetic nerves (however, because cholinergic sympathetic nerves had not yet been discovered, there was a great debate over the mechanism of perspiration induced by the parasympathetic nerve stimulant pilocarpine and the presence or absence of dual innervation of the sweat glands by sympathetic and parasympathetic nerves, in a fashion similar to that in other organs). In 1875, Goltz reported that electrical stimulation of the sciatic nerve of cats caused perspiration on the pads of the rear feet [1]. Subsequently, Luchsing-

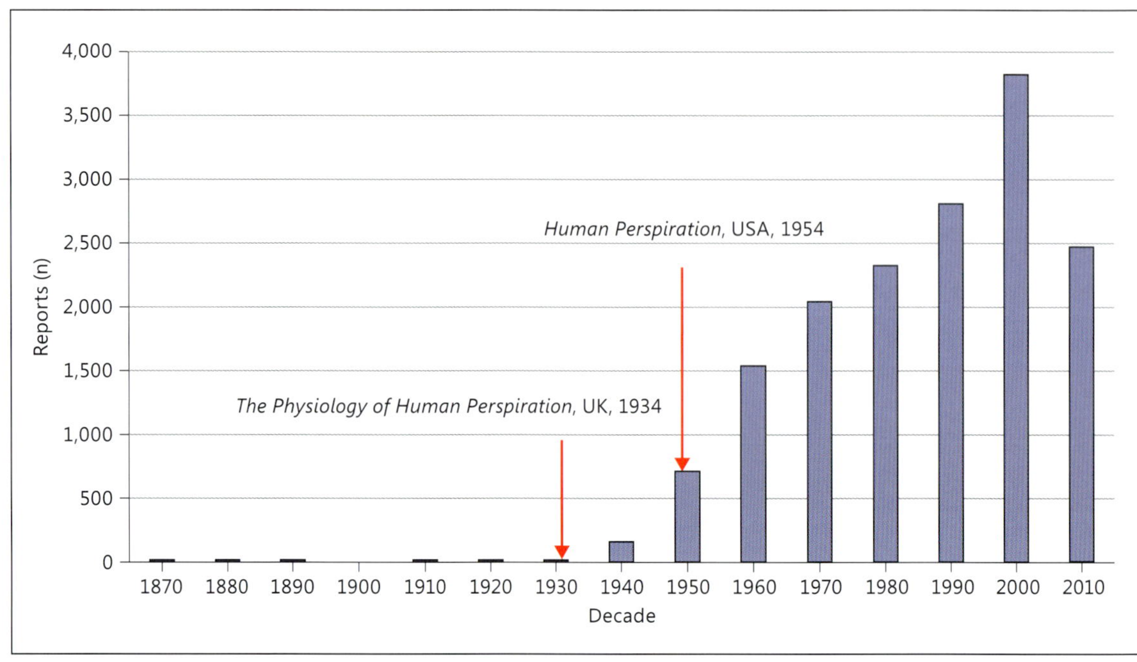

Fig. 1. The number of reports on perspiration increased sharply in the 1950s.

er, who is called the father of studies on the physiology of perspiration, and others reported that although perspiration disappears when the sympathetic nerve trunk is extracted, perspiration takes place in response to atropine, and electrical stimulation of the sciatic nerve causes mild perspiration despite extraction of the sympathetic nerve trunk, demonstrating dual innervation of the sweat glands. Meanwhile, Langley and colleagues denied dual innervation of the sweat glands and insisted on the concept of single innervation by the sympathetic nerves [1].

However, the results of studies on the physiology of perspiration were minimally utilized clinically. That is, there was no impetus whatsoever to diagnose a responsible lesion or a causative disease based on patterns of perspiration abnormalities. Moreover, clinicians' interests were concentrated on excessive perspiration alone, and decreased perspiration was not even studied in clinical settings. The first reason was that perspiration abnormalities were macroscopically examined clinically, such that decreased perspiration was not easily recognized. The second reason was that clinical research on the autonomic nervous system was targeted as an 'autonomic nervous system imbalance' showing increased autonomic function, and the presence of autonomic failure syndrome showing decreased autonomic function was not recognized. However, in 1928, Victor Minor [2], a Russian neurologist, established a qualitative method of determining perspiration sites using the starch-iodine method, and Dr. Kuno, a professor of Manchuria Medical College, reported a study on human perspiration over the whole body using the ventilated capsule method in 1934 and 1954 [3, 4]. This enabled both qualitative and quantitative determination of the amount of perspiration over the whole body, markedly advancing our understanding of the physiology of perspiration. The number of reports on perspiration increased sharply thereafter, to over 200 in the 1940s and then over 700 in the 1950s after the discovery of the ventilated capsule methods which can measure human perspiration over the whole body in 1934 and 1954 [3, 4] (fig. 1).

Maturation Stage of Perspiration Research

Clinical studies of perspiration abnormalities require easy and simple tests to objectively determine distributions of perspiration abnormalities. Thus, it is no exaggeration to say that clinical perspiration research blossomed with the invention of the Minor method (the starch-iodine method). Using his starch-iodine method, Minor also reported that thermal sweating occurs at hairy areas over the whole body, whereas emotional sweating occurs at the palms and soles [2]. On behalf of Minor, Guttmann and List [5], two German brain surgeons, established the usefulness of the Minor method and spread its use to the United Kingdom and the United States. They introduced the Minor method to research sweat nerve conduction pathways.

Immediately after co-writing the above paper, List was exiled to the US; he continued to study perspiration using the Minor method in the US and co-wrote and published a book entitled *Sweat Secretion in Man* with Peet in the period from 1938 to 1939. This paper was cited as a key article in most English publications on clinical perspiration research in the 1940s. Meanwhile, based on clues obtained using the Minor method, Guttmann [6] developed the quinizarin method in 1937. The major turning point in clinical research on perspiration was the discovery that sweat nerves are cholinergic sympathetic nerves and the establishment of a diagnostic theory based on the results of sweating induced by drugs such as acetylcholine and pilocarpine. However, the Minor method made it possible for the first time to prove that the sweating nerves in humans are cholinergic.

Sweating nerves were proven to be cholinergic by Rothman and Coon [7], at the Department of Dermatology, University of Chicago, and Hyndman and Wolkin [8], at the Department of Brain Surgery, Iowa State University, in the US. Rothman and Coon studied the perspiration reaction in humans when receiving an intracutaneous injection of acetylcholine using the Minor method and reported that perspiration induced by acetylcholine occurs more extensively in the area where the drug directly infiltrated. After the 1940s, there was a rapid increase in the number of papers on the Minor method in the UK and the US, and modified Minor methods were developed sequentially. From the second half of the 1950s, reports describing perspiration abnormalities in clinical cases using the Minor method (or modified techniques) started to accumulate. However, most of these clinical reports were on pathologies showing decreased perspiration, not excessive perspiration.

With the appearance of the Minor method, there was a major shift in the theme of clinical research on perspiration from excessive to decreased perspiration. This is because the Minor method is essentially a qualitative test, suitable for the detection of decreased perspiration rather than excessive perspiration. As we all know, methods developed without relevance to the Minor method have often been used in perspiration research in recent years. These include the capsule ventilation method, sympathetic skin response, and microneurography. However, the distribution of perspiration abnormalities cannot be studied in detail with these methods, and the Minor method (or modifications thereof) is still the only way to determine the presence of sweating abnormalities.

Dr. Yasu Kuno published papers on measuring the amount of perspiration over the whole body using the ventilated capsule method while he was a professor at Manchuria Medical College,

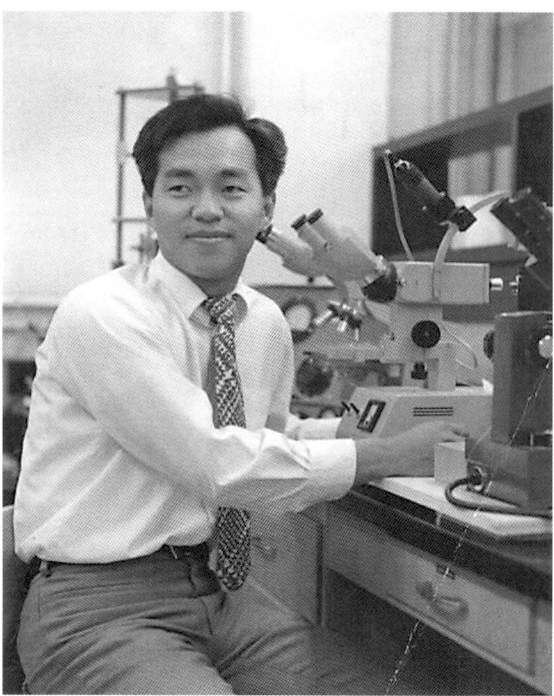

Fig. 2. A photograph of Dr. Sato.

making it possible to quantitatively determine the amount of perspiration over the entire body surface [3, 4]. The ventilated capsule for sweat measurement is placed at the measurement site; air (nitrogen) is sent to the capsule to cause the sweat to evaporate, and the amount of water in the air is detected to measure the amount of perspiration. This enables measurement of the amounts of trace moisture such as with emotional sweating [3, 4]. In recent years, a simple ventilated capsule for measuring the amount of perspiration using a humidity sensor was developed and is now used to study many diseases [9]. Thereafter, Dr. Kuno continued to study different innervations involved in emotional sweating and thermal sweating, as well as cholinergic sweat glands, albeit those innervated by sympathetic nerves, while as a professor at Nagoya University, which built the foundation of the present study of the physiology of perspiration. He was twice a candidate for the Nobel Prize, nominated in Physiology and Medicine [3, 4].

The development of these qualitative and quantitative methods to determine the amount of perspiration in humans dramatically advanced perspiration research and clinical research on perspiration [2–4]. In the maturation stage, there were advances in the study of eccrine sweat glands, the sweating organs. In particular, the accomplishments of Dr. Kenzo Sato (fig. 2), a professor at the University of Iowa, had the greatest impact on the advancement of studies on the physiology of perspiration. After graduating from Hokkaido University School of Medicine in 1964, Dr. Sato studied at the University of Oregon in 1967, where he started his research on sweat glands at the laboratories of professors Dobson and Lobitz. He then established a method of analyzing the perspiration function of isolated sweat glands in vitro at the Department of Dermatology and the Department of Physiology at Radboud University Nijmegen (the Netherlands) from 1970 to 1971 [10]. He then returned to the US and energetically studied the physiology of perspiration at the Department of Dermatology, University of Iowa, led by Professor John Strauss, from 1978 to 1997. With this electrophysiological analysis using an in vitro experimental system focusing on a single sweat gland by the patch clamp method, he demonstrated, for the first time, the presence of not only the choline receptor, but also adrenergic α- and β-receptors and the mechanism of sweat secretion by Na-K-2Cl cotransport, K-, Cl channels, and the Na-pump [10–12]. Dr. Sato reported the results of many analyses of the secretion function of sweat glands and analyses of the pathology of cystic fibrosis, publishing over 100 reports, primarily in prestigious journals of basic research such as the *Journal of Clinical Investigation*, the *Journal of Physiology*, and the *American Journal of Physiology* [10–12].

What these two great researchers, who advanced our knowledge of the physiology of per-

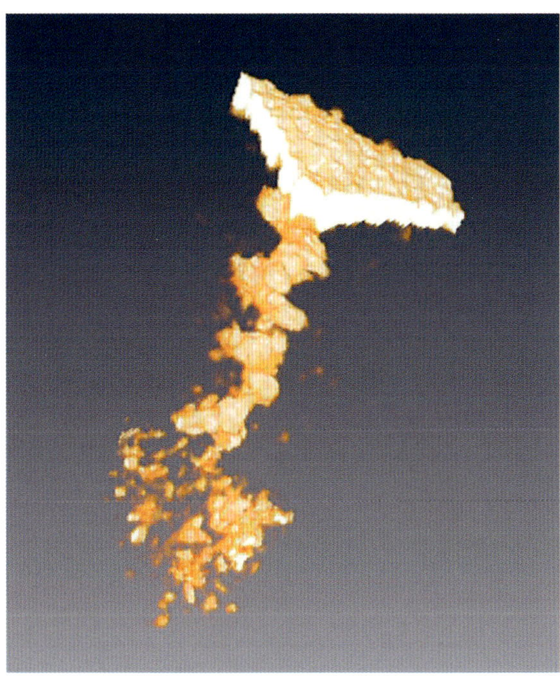

Fig. 3. Three-dimensional analysis of the sweat glands in the stratum corneum of the skin.

spiration historically, share in common is that they established Japanese-style research methods not by mimicking researchers from Western countries, but by applying their own insights. Furthermore, their research bases were overseas.

Development Stage of Perspiration Research

Perspiration research entered the development stage in the 2000s; it has since been elucidated that perspiration has not only a temperature-regulating function and a non-slip function for the hands and feet, but also a natural immunity function to protect the body from bacteria, with an antimicrobial peptide called dermcidin contained in sweat [13]. Moreover, it has been reported that obstruction of the sweat glands plays a major role in the onset of disorders such as parapsoriasis, lichen planus, and lichen amyloidosis [14, 15], and that *Malassezia* is an allergen in sweat, a factor exacerbating atopic dermatitis and cholinergic urticaria [16], making perspiration abnormalities possible causes of many allergic skin disorders. Furthermore, the sweat glands were found to play numerous roles, including storage of stem cells to replenish epidermal cells at the time of thermal burns and moisture retention to replenish moisture in the stratum corneum of the skin.

In our department, we analyze the 3-dimensional structures of sweat glands in disorders such as hyperhidrosis, using high-speed en face optical coherence tomography which can visualize the sweat glands dynamically and 3-dimensionally. Optical coherence tomography provides 3-dimensional imaging using optical interference; it visualizes the structures of biological tissues under the epidermis at high resolution and can display the structure of the sweat ducts in the stratum corneum and the epidermis (fig. 3) [17]. It has now been demonstrated that in patients with primary focal hyperhidrosis, the amount of sweat present in the sweat ducts in the stratum corneum is greater than normal, as is the frequency of opening and closing of the sweat pores, and pore opening time is also longer. Three-dimensional analysis of the sweat glands is likely to unravel novel pathologies of skin disorders.

References

1 Tamura T: A history of perspiration research. Jpn J Perspiration Res 2015;22:69–72.
2 Minor V: Ein neues Verfahren zu der klinischen Untersuchung der Schweissabsonderung. Dtsch Z Nervenheilk 1928;101:302–308.
3 Kuno Y: The Physiology of Human Perspiration. London, Churchill, 1934.
4 Kuno Y: Human Perspiration. Springfield, Charles C. Thomas, 1954.
5 Guttmann L, List CF: Zur Topik und Pathophysiologie der Schweisssekretion. Z ges Neurol Psychiatr 1928;116:504–536.

6 Guttmann L: Die Schweisssekretion des Menschen in ihren Beziehungen zum Nervensystem. Z ges Neurol Psychiatr 1931;135:1–48.
7 Rothman S, Coon JM: Axon reflex responses to acetyl choline in the skin. J Invest Dermatol 1940;3:79–97.
8 Hyndman OR, Wolkin J: The pilocarpine sweating test I. A valid indicator in differentiation of preganglionic and postganglionic sympathectomy. Arch Neurol Psychiatr 1941;45:992–1006.
9 Yokozeki H, Katayama I, Nishioka K, Kinoshita M, Nishiyama S: The role of metal allergy and local hyperhidrosis in the pathogenesis of pompholyx. J Dermatol 1992;19:964–967.
10 Sato K, Sato F: Phamacologic responsiveness if isolated single eccrine sweat glands. Am J Physiol 1981;240:R44–R51.
11 Sato K, Sato F: Defective beta adrenergic response of cystic fibrosis sweat glands in vivo and in vitro. J Clin Invest 1984; 73:1763–1771.
12 Sato K, Kang WH, Saga K, Sato KT: Biology of the eccrine sweat gland. I: mechanism of sweat secretion. J Am Acad Dermatol 1989;20:537–565.
13 Schittek B, Hipfel R, Sauer B, Bauer J, Kalbacher H, Stevanovic S, Schirle M, Schroeder K, Blin N, Meier F, Rassner G, Garbe C: Dermcidin: a novel human antibiotic peptide secreted by sweat glands. Nat Immunol 2001;2:1133–1137.
14 Hayakawa J, Mizukawa Y, Kurata M, Shiohara T: A syringotropic variant of cutaneous sarcoidosis: presentation of 3 cases exhibiting defective sweating responses. J Am Acad Dermatol 2013;68: 1016–1021.
15 Mizukawa Y, Ikehara Y, Nishihara S, Shiohara T, Narimatsu H: An immunohistochemical study of beta 1,4-galactosyltransferase in human skin tissue. J Dermatol Sci 1999;20:183–190.
16 Hiragun T, Ishii K, Hiragun M, Suzuki H, Kan T, Mihara S, Yanase Y, Bartels J, Schröder JM, Hide M: Fungal protein MGL_1304 in sweat is an allergen for atopic dermatitis patients. J Allergy Clin Immunol 2013;132:608–615.
17 Ohmi M, Tanigawa M, Wada Y, Haruna M: Dynamic analysis for mental sweating of a group of eccrine sweat glands on a human fingertip by optical coherence tomography. Skin Res Technol 2012;18: 378–383.

Prof. Hiroo Yokozeki
Department of Dermatology
Graduate School of Medical and Dental Sciences
Tokyo Medical and Dental University
1-5-45 Yushima, Bunkyo-ku
Tokyo 113-8519 (Japan)
E-Mail 3064derm@tmd.ac.jp

Yokozeki H, Murota H, Katayama I (eds): Perspiration Research.
Curr Probl Dermatol. Basel, Karger, 2016, vol 51, pp 7–10 (DOI: 10.1159/000446753)

Classification of Systemic and Localized Sweating Disorders

Yuichiro Ohshima • Yasuhiko Tamada

Department of Dermatology, Aichi Medical University School of Medicine, Nagakute, Japan

Abstract

Hyperhidrosis can be subdivided into generalized hyperhidrosis, with increased sweating over the entire body, and focal hyperhidrosis, in which the excessive sweating is restricted to specific parts of the body. Generalized hyperhidrosis may be either primary (idiopathic) or secondary. Secondary generalized hyperhidrosis may be caused by infections such as tuberculosis, hyperthyroidism, endocrine and metabolic disturbances such as pheochromocytoma, neurological disorders, or drugs. Focal hyperhidrosis may also be primary (idiopathic) or secondary. Frey's syndrome is one form of secondary focal hyperhidrosis that occurs during eating together with reddening of the area in front of the ear following parotid gland surgery or injury. Primary focal hyperhidrosis is particularly common on the palms and soles of the feet, in the axilla, and on the head. Anhidrosis may be either congenital/genetic or acquired. Some of the most typical forms of congenital/genetic anhidrosis include hypohidrotic ectodermal dysplasia, congenital insensitivity to pain and anhidrosis, and Fabry disease. Acquired anhidrosis is classified as secondary anhidrosis, which may be due to an underlying disorder such as a neurological disorder, an endocrine or metabolic disturbance, or the effect of drugs, or idiopathic anhidrosis for which the pathology, cause, and mechanism are unknown. Idiopathic anhidrosis is classified into acquired idiopathic generalized anhidrosis (AIGA), idiopathic segmental anhidrosis, and Ross syndrome. AIGA is divided into three categories according to differences in the site of disturbance: (1) sudomotor neuropathy, (2) idiopathic pure sudomotor failure, and (3) sweat gland failure.

Hyperhidrosis

Hyperhidrosis represents sweating that exceeds the amount necessary to control body temperature, to the extent that it interferes with activities of daily living or work [1]. This pathology can be subdivided into generalized hyperhidrosis, with increased sweating over the entire body, and focal hyperhidrosis, in which the excessive sweating is restricted to specific parts of the body. Generalized hyperhidrosis may be either primary (idiopathic) or secondary, occurring together with other conditions. Secondary generalized hyperhidrosis may be caused by infections such as tuberculosis, hyperthyroidism, endocrine and meta-

Table 1. Causes of secondary generalized hyperhidrosis

Infection	Tuberculosis, bacterial endocarditis, liver abscess, cholangitis, pyelonephritis, sepsis
Endocrine disorder	Hyperthyroidism, acromegaly, pheochromocytoma, menopausal symptoms
Metabolic disorder	Diabetes, obesity, insulinoma
Circulatory disorder	Congestive heart failure, orthostatic hypotension
Malignant tumor	Malignant lymphoma, malignant tumor
Connective tissue disease	Systemic lupus erythematosus
Neurological disorder	Cerebrovascular disturbance, brain tumor, Parkinson's disease, Shy-Drager syndrome
Drug-induced side effect	Psychotropics, sleep-inducing drugs, nonsteroidal anti-inflammatories, steroids

bolic disturbances such as pheochromocytoma, neurological disorders, or drugs. In terms of neurological disorders, abnormalities of the cerebral cortex can either elevate or reduce sweating function. In the event of increased sweating on the paralyzed side after cerebral infarction, hyperhidrosis may also be induced by damage to the diencephalon, which contains the hypothalamus, the structure responsible for the central control of body temperature, or by autonomic nervous impairment due to spinal cord damage (table 1). Focal hyperhidrosis may also be primary (idiopathic) or secondary. Frey's syndrome is one form of secondary focal hyperhidrosis that occurs during eating together with reddening of the area in front of the ear following parotid gland surgery or injury. This is attributed to damage to the parasympathetic innervations of the nerves that govern sweating [2].

The diagnostic criteria for primary focal hyperhidrosis have been defined by Hornberger et al. [3] as the presence of localized excessive sweating with no obvious cause for at least 6 months that meets at least 2 of the following 6 symptoms:

1 Bilateral and relatively symmetric
2 Impairment of daily activities
3 Frequency of at least 1 episode/week
4 Age at onset <25 years
5 Positive family history
6 Cessation of focal sweating during sleep

Primary focal hyperhidrosis is particularly common on the palms and soles of the feet, in the axilla, and on the head. Prevalence and age at onset in Japan are 5.33% and 13.8 years for the palms, 2.79% and 15.9 years for the soles of the feet, 5.75% and 19.5 years for the axilla, and 4.7% and 21.2 years for the head, respectively. These rates are higher than those reported for America [4].

Anhidrosis

Anhidrosis refers to the absence (or reduction) of sweating even under conditions that would normally promote it (exercise, heat, or high humidity). Anhidrosis may be either congenital/genetic or acquired [5]. Some of the most typical forms of congenital/genetic anhidrosis include hypohidrotic ectodermal dysplasia, congenital insensitivity to pain and anhidrosis, and Fabry disease.

Hypohidrotic ectodermal dysplasia is a rare genetic disorder characterized by the faulty development of the ectodermal structure, resulting most notably in anhidrosis/hypohidrosis (lack of sweat glands), hypotrichosis (sparseness of scalp and body hair), and hypodontia (congenital absence of teeth) [6, 7]. This condition is usually an X-linked recessive disorder affecting predominantly males [8].

Congenital insensitivity to pain and anhidrosis is characterized by autosomal recessive inheritance with recurrent episodes of unexplained fever, failure to thrive, insensitivity to pain, self-mutilation, and mild mental retardation. The lack of pain sensation often results in severe oral mutilation. Bite wounds have been reported to cause

Table 2. Classification of acquired anhidrosis

Type	Disorder
Idiopathic	AIGA Idiopathic segmental anhidrosis Ross syndrome
Secondary	
Sympathetic nerve disturbance	Central: Horner syndrome, brainstem damage Peripheral: polyneuritis, Sjögren syndrome
Associated with skin disorder	Miliaria Chronic inflammatory dermatitis (seborrheic dermatitis, atopic dermatitis) Keratotic disorders (psoriasis, lichen planus, Darier disease) Ichthyosis Atrophic lesions (scleroderma, lichen sclerosus et atrophicus, chronic radiodermatitis, xeroderma pigmentosum)
Endocrine or metabolic disturbance	Hypothalamic disturbance (diabetes insipidus, Simmonds' disease, Addison's disease) Hypothyroidism Severe dehydration
Drug-induced	Atropine, scopolamine, tetraethylammonium, hexamethonium, etc.

laceration and ulceration of the tongue, lips, and other oral mucosa. Tooth luxation and severe dental attrition have also been observed. Other problems include chronic bone and joint infections [9, 10]. Despite the presence of normal sweat glands, the absence of postganglionic sympathetic fibers innervating the sweat glands means that no sweating occurs. The genetic mutation is in the gene encoding the neurotrophic tyrosine kinase receptor *(NTRK1)* [11].

Fabry disease is a rare X-linked lysosomal storage disorder characterized by deficiency of the lysosomal enzyme α-galactosidase A. This results in systemic accumulation of globotriaosylceramide and related glycosphingolipids in the lysosomes of cells throughout the body. Early symptoms in classically affected male and female patients include angiokeratoma, anhidrosis, neuropathic pain, gastrointestinal symptoms, and microalbuminuria. Progressive renal failure, heart failure, and stroke generally occur later in life [12]. Globotriaosylceramide accumulates in the endocrine regions of sweat glands, and anhidrosis is evident [13].

Acquired anhidrosis is classified as secondary anhidrosis, which may be due to an underlying disorder such as a neurological disorder, an endocrine or metabolic disturbance, or the effect of drugs, or idiopathic anhidrosis for which the pathology, cause, and mechanism are unknown (table 2). Of the different types of idiopathic anhidrosis, the absence of sweating in acquired idiopathic generalized anhidrosis (AIGA) extends over almost the entire body and is defined as 'an acquired reduction in sweating without any obvious cause and no autonomic or neurological abnormalities other than impaired sweating' [5]. This impairment of sweating, which plays an important role in controlling body temperature, means that the core temperature in the patient can easily rise during exercise or under hot conditions. AIGA is therefore distinguished from disorders such as idiopathic segmental anhidrosis [14] and Ross syndrome [15], in which the absence of sweating is distributed segmentally. AIGA is divided into three categories according to differences in the site of disturbance: (1) sudomotor neuropathy, in which only the sudomotor nerves of the sympathetic nervous system are disturbed, (2) idiopathic pure sudomotor failure, arising from acetylcholine receptor abnormalities, and (3) sweat gland failure, arising from abnormalities in the sweat glands. The core clinical features of idiopathic pure sudomotor failure are: (1) predominant involvement of young males, (2) strong association with pain or abnormal sensation and cholinergic urticaria, (3) preservation of emotional sweating, (4) absence of organic skin lesions, (5) absence of dysautonomias other than anhidrosis, (6) complete response to steroid therapy, (7) possibility of spontaneous remission, and (8) high levels of immunoglobulin E [5, 16].

References

1 Sato K, Kang WH, Saga K, Sato KT: Biology of sweat glands and its disorders. II. Disorders of sweat gland function. J Am Acad Dermatol 1989;20:713–726.
2 Drummond PD: Mechanism of gustatory flushing in Frey's syndrome. Clin Auton Res 2002;12:144–146.
3 Hornberger J, Grimes K, Naumann M, et al: Recognition, diagnosis, and treatment of primary focal hyperhidrosis. J Am Acad Dermatol 2004;51:274–286.
4 Fujimoto T, Kawahara K, Yokozeki H: Epidemiological study and considerations of focal hyperhidrosis in Japan: from questionnaire analysis. J Dermatol 2013;40:886–890.
5 Nakazato Y, Tamura N, Ohkuma A, et al: Idiopathic pure sudomotor failure: anhidrosis due to deficits in cholinergic transmission. Neurology 2004;63:1476–1480.
6 Soloman LH, Kener EJ: The ectodermal dysplasia. Arch Dermatol 1980;116:295–299.
7 Weech AA: Hereditary ectodermal dysplasia of the anhidrotic type. A report of two cases. Am J Dis Child 1929;37:766–790.
8 Reed WB, Lopez DA, Lauding B: Clinical spectrum of anhidrotic ectodermal dysplasia. Arch Dermatol 1970;102:134–143.
9 Amano A, Akiyama S, Ikeda M, Morisaki I: Oral manifestations of hereditary sensory and autonomic neuropathy type IV. Congenital insensitivity to pain with anhidrosis. Oral Surg Oral Med Oral Pathol Oral Radiol Endod 1998;86:425–431.
10 Paduano S, Iodice G, Farella M, Silva R, Michelotti A: Orthodontic treatment and management of limited mouth opening and oral lesions in a patient with congenital insensitivity to pain: case report. J Oral Rehabil 2009;36:71–78.
11 Indo Y, Tsuruta M, Hayashida Y, et al: Mutations in the TRKA/NGF receptor gene in patients with congenital insensitivity to pain with anhidrosis. Nat Genet 1996;13:485–488.
12 Arends M, Hollak CE, Biegstraaten M: Quality of life in patients with Fabry disease: a systematic review of the literature. Orphanet J Rare Dis 2015;10:77.
13 Desnick RJ, Ioannou YA, Eng CM, et al: α-Galactosidase A deficiency: Fabry disease; in Scriver CR, Beaudet AL, Sly WS, Valle D: The Metabolic and Molecular Bases of Inherited Disease, ed 7. New York, McGraw-Hill, 1995, pp 2741–2785.
14 Nakazato Y, Tamura N, Ohkuma A, Yoshimaru K, Shimazu K: Thermogram of idiopathic segmental anhidrosis. Neurology 2005;64:2084.
15 Ross AT: Progressive selective sudomotor denervation. Neurology 1958;8:809–817.
16 Ohshima Y, Yanagishita T, Ito K, et al: Treatment of patients with acquired idiopathic generalized anhidrosis. Br J Dermatol 2013;168:430–432.

Yuichiro Ohshima
Department of Dermatology
Aichi Medical University School of Medicine
Nagakute 480-1195 (Japan)
E-Mail y45123@aichi-med-u.ac.jp

Yokozeki H, Murota H, Katayama I (eds): Perspiration Research.
Curr Probl Dermatol. Basel, Karger, 2016, vol 51, pp 11–21 (DOI: 10.1159/000446754)

New Findings on the Mechanism of Perspiration Including Aquaporin-5 Water Channel

Risako Inoue
Department of Dermatology, Graduate School of Medical and Dental Sciences, Tokyo Medical and Dental University, Tokyo, Japan

Abstract
Aquaporin-5 (AQP5) is a member of the water channel protein family. Although AQP5 has been shown to be present in sweat glands, the presence or absence of regulated intracellular translocation of AQP5 in sweat glands remains to be determined. In this article, recent findings on AQP5 in sweat glands are presented. (1) Immunoreactive AQP5 was detected in the apical membranes and the intercellular canaliculi of secretory coils, and in the basolateral membranes of the clear cells in human eccrine sweat glands. (2) AQP5 rapidly concentrated at the apical membranes during sweating in mouse sweat glands. (3) Treatment of human AQP5-expressing Madin-Darby canine kidney cells with calcium ionophore A23187 resulted in a twofold increase in the AQP5 level in the apical membranes within 5 min. (4) Anoctamin-1, a calcium-activated chloride channel was detected in the apical membranes and it completely colocalized with AQP5 in the apical membranes in mouse sweat glands. AQP5 may be involved in sweating and its translocation may help to increase the water permeability of the apical membranes of sweat glands. AQP5 is a potential target molecule for the design of a sweat-modulating drug.

Secretion of fluid is the principal function of eccrine sweat glands. An eccrine sweat gland is a single tubular structure consisting of a secretory portion and a ductal portion. In the secretory portion, primary fluid, i.e. primary sweat, is secreted into the lumen by active salt transport followed by movement of water, and the fluid transits through the duct where salt reabsorption occurs [1, 2]. It is expected that regulation of fluid movement is important in this process.

Aquaporins (AQPs) are a family of integral membrane channel proteins that allow the rapid movement of water across the plasma membrane. Thirteen members of the AQP family (AQP0–AQP12) have been identified in mammals to date, and these proteins are expressed in various fluid-transporting epithelia with a distinct tissue-specific pattern [3]. There have been a few reports regarding the presence of AQP5 in sweat glands [4–9]. In this article, new findings which have been published in recent years on the role of AQP5 in sweat secretion are described [10].

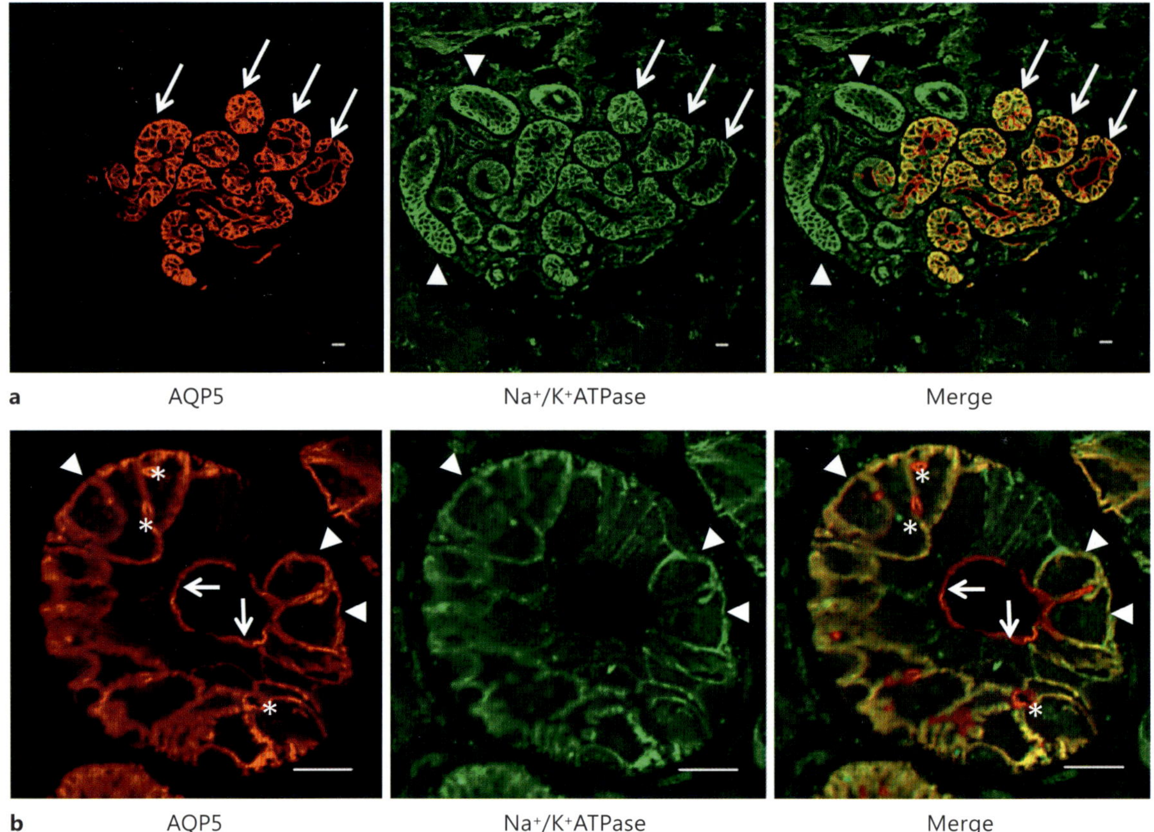

Fig. 1. Immunohistochemical analysis of AQP5 localization in human eccrine sweat glands. **a** Representative double-immunofluorescent staining of AQP5 (red) and Na^+/K^+ATPase (green) in a paraffin section of a human eccrine sweat gland. Immunoreactive AQP5 was detected in cells of the secretory portion of the gland (arrows), but not in duct cells (arrowheads). **b** Close-up images of the secretary coil of a human eccrine sweat gland. Immunoreactive AQP5 was detected in the apical membranes (arrows) and in the intercellular canaliculi (asterisks), and did not colocalize with Na^+/K^+ATPase in these areas. AQP5 was also detected in the basolateral membranes of the clear cells (arrowheads) where it did colocalize with Na^+/K^+ATPase. Bar = 10 μm.

Immunohistochemical Analysis of Aquaporin-5 Localization in Human Eccrine Sweat Glands

To determine the cellular localization of AQP5 in human eccrine sweat glands, our group immunohistochemically analyzed paraffin sections of healthy human skin using anti-AQP5 antibody (ab93230, Abcam). In addition, anti-Na^+/K^+ATPase antibody (sc-21712, Sigma-Aldrich) was used for visualizing the morphology of the eccrine sweat gland (fig. 1). Immunoreactive AQP5 was detected in cells in the secretory portion of the eccrine sweat gland, but not in duct cells, whereas immunoreactive Na^+/K^+ATPase was detected in cells of both the secretory portion and the duct. Sweat gland duct cells showed strong Na^+/K^+ATPase labeling at their basolateral plasma membranes as previously [11, 12] and subsequently [13] reported, whereas cells in the secretory portion showed relatively weak labeling at their basolateral plasma membranes (fig. 1a). AQP5 was detected in the apical membranes (fig. 1b, arrows) of cells in the secretory portion as well as in the intercellular canaliculi (fig. 1b, asterisks), and this AQP5 staining did not colocalize with Na^+/K^+ATPase staining. In addition, AQP5 was also detected in the basolateral membranes of the clear cells (fig. 1b, arrowheads). Analysis of different specimens of healthy skin from several patients using two other anti-AQP5 antibodies (sc-9890 and sc-28628, Santa Cruz Biotechnology) indicated almost exactly the same distribution of AQP5 as that shown in figure 1a and b. AQP5 was not detected in other components of the skin, including the epidermis, sebaceous glands, and hair follicles (data not shown).

Aquaporin-5 Translocates from the Nonapical Region to the Apical Membranes in Cells of Mouse Sweat Glands under Sweating Conditions

AQP2 is a water channel in the collecting ducts of the kidney that translocates from intracellular membranes to plasma membranes in response to vasopressin [14–16]. AQP5 has 63% identity to AQP2 [17] and was shown to translocate from the cytoplasm to the apical membranes in cells of rat salivary glands by stimulation with M_3 muscarinic and α_1-adrenergic agonists [18, 19], and in cells of rat parotid glands with cevimeline [20]. However, there has been no report regarding AQP5 translocation in cells of sweat glands. Therefore, we assessed changes in the subcellular localization of AQP5 in sweat glands during sweating in mice (C57BL6/J). Since it was difficult to investigate the mechanism of AQP5 translocation in human tissues, we used mouse tissues for this investigation.

Whether the mice were sweating or not through their paws was determined using a modified Minor method; mouse paws were painted with 3% iodine in ethanol, coated with 80% starch solution in olive oil, and observed. To obtain nonsweating mice, we intraperitoneally anesthetized the mice. To make the mice sweat, we simply held the mice in our hands without anesthesia. We chose this method because more spots were observed on the paws of the held mice than the mice given a sweating agent such as pilocarpine or acetylcholine.

In the control anesthetized mice, spots corresponding to sweat secretion were scarcely observed on the paws (fig. 2a). In the sweating group, spots appear on their paws soon after holding (fig. 2b). After confirming that the mice were in a nonsweating or sweating condition, the paws were removed and processed for immunofluorescence using rabbit monoclonal anti-AQP5 (ab93230, Abcam) for the primary antibody. Under nonsweating condition, AQP5 was detected in the apical membranes of secretory cells in the mouse sweat glands, and was diffusely localized in the nonapical region (fig. 3a, b). Under sweating condition, almost all AQP5 staining was detected in the apical membranes (fig. 3c, d). This apical accumulation of AQP5 was also confirmed in pilocarpine-induced sweating. The fluorescent intensity in the apical AQP5 in the cross-section of the coils was significantly increased from 60 ± 7.7% (n = 15) under nonsweating condition to 91 ± 6.0% (n = 15) under sweating condition (mean ± SD, $p < 0.01$). These data suggest that a certain amount of AQP5 translocated from the nonapical region to the apical membranes during sweating.

Transfected Human Aquaporin-5 Is Located at Both the Apical and Basolateral Membranes of Madin-Darby Canine Kidney Cells

To further investigate AQP5 cellular localization and translocation, we generated Madin-Darby canine kidney (MDCK) cell lines stably expressing nontagged human AQP5 (hAQP5). The transfected hAQP5 was not tagged since some tag sequences are known to affect the cellular localization of AQP5 [21]. We selected nine clones from these transfected cells based on Western blotting of AQP5 protein expression (fig. 4a). Of these clones, clone No. 6, which showed a high level of AQP5 expression, and a mixture of clones Nos. 4, 7, and 9, which was used to avoid the effect of clonal variation on the results, were selected for further experiments. A cell-side-specific biotinylation assay showed that hAQP5 was present at both the apical and basolateral membranes of these cells (fig. 4b), which was consistent with the immunohistochemical localization of AQP5 in human eccrine sweat glands in vivo (fig. 1).

There must be high water permeability in both apical and basolateral plasma membranes for tight epithelia to be highly permeable to water. In kidney collecting ducts, there are AQP3 and AQP4 in the basolateral plasma membranes, which make the membranes constitutively permeable to water. The trafficking of AQP2 to the apical membranes is the key machinery to increase transepithelial water permeability by vasopressin signaling. It is possible to speculate that basolateral AQP5 in sweat glands may have the same role as AQP3 and AQP4 in the collecting ducts.

Human Aquaporin-5 Translocates from the Cytoplasm to the Apical Membranes by Treatment with Calcium Ionophore

In rat parotid glands, the interaction of acetylcholine with M_3 muscarinic receptors and of norepinephrine with α_1-adrenergic receptors stimulates salivary secretion by inducing an elevation of intracellular calcium concentration and the translocation of rat AQP5 from the intracellular mem-

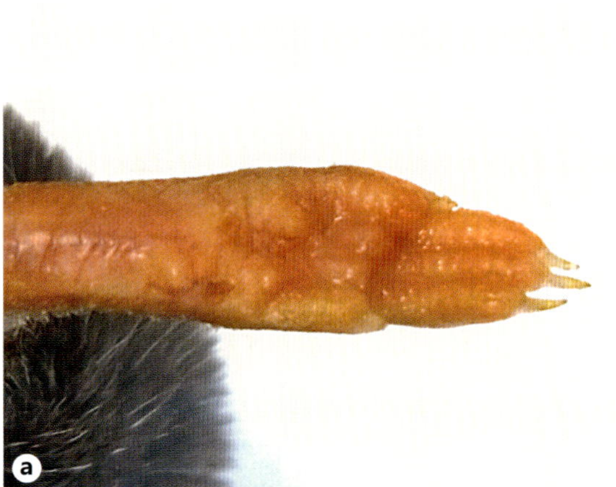

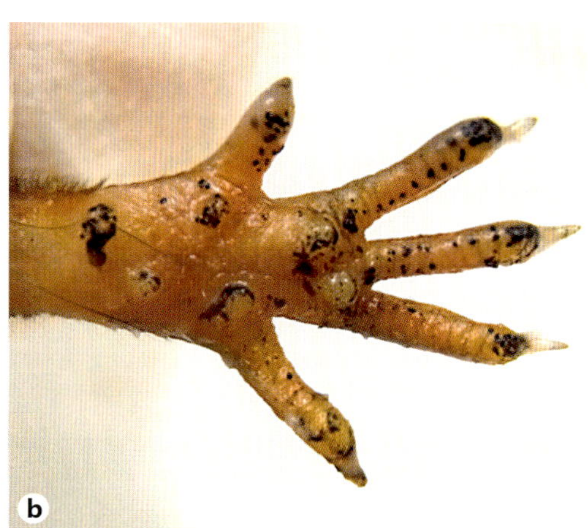

Fig. 2. Confirmation of nonsweating/sweating of mice through their paws. Representative photographs of paws of nonsweating/sweating mice are shown. **a** No spot corresponding to sweat secretion was apparent on the paw of an anesthetized mouse. **b** Numerous spots were observed on the paw of a mouse which was held in the hand without anesthesia (5-min holding).

Fig. 3. AQP5 translocation from the nonapical region to the apical membranes of cells in mouse sweat glands. **a–d** Immunofluorescent staining of AQP5 localization in paraffin sections of a representative mouse sweat gland under nonsweating or sweating conditions. **a**, **b** Under nonsweating condition, immunoreactive AQP5 was detected in the apical membranes as well as in the nonapical region of the secretory cells. **c**, **d** Under sweating condition, almost all immunoreactive AQP5 was detected in the apical membranes. Bar = 10 μm. DIC = Differential interference contrast.

(For figure see next page.)

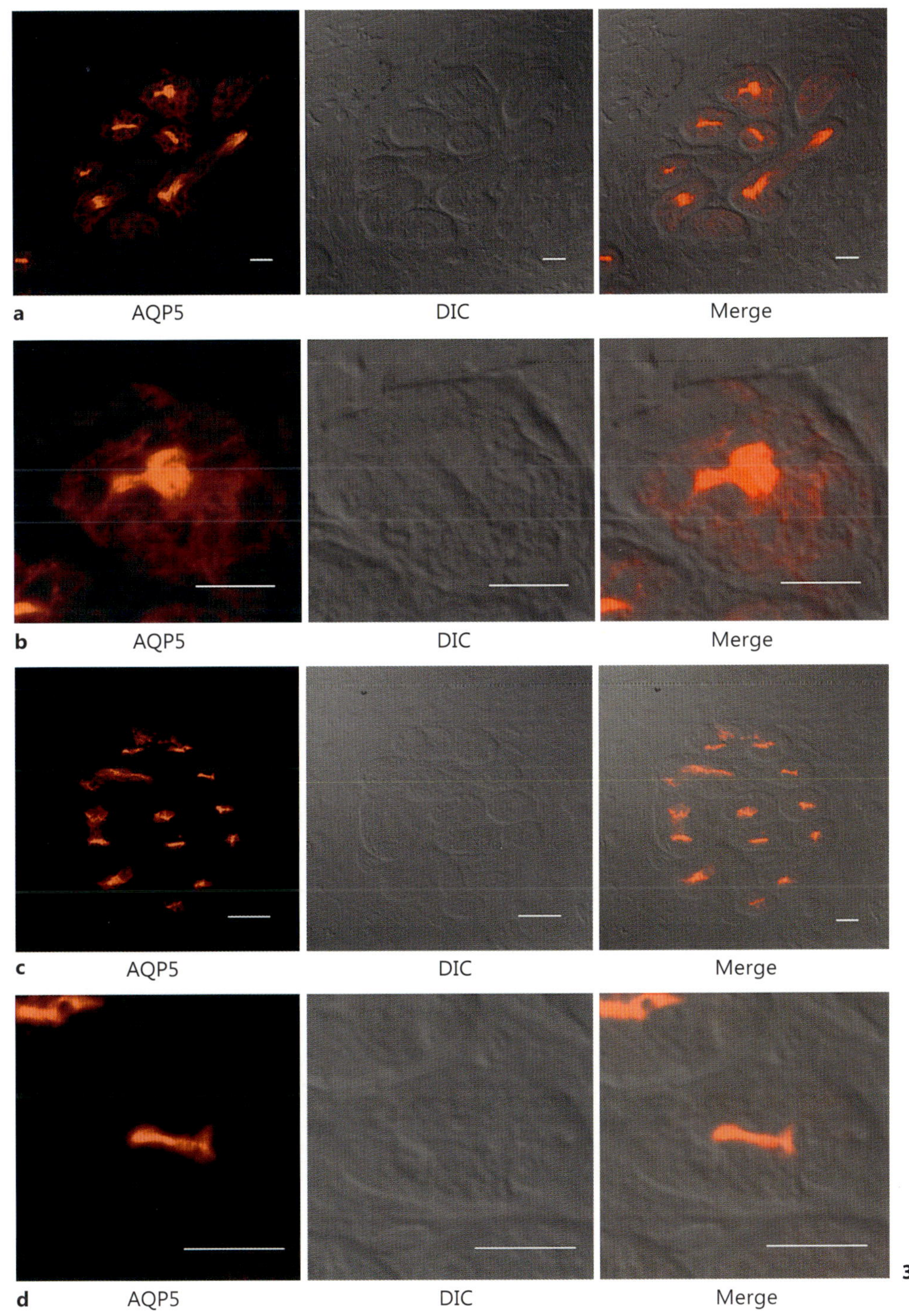
a
AQP5
DIC
Merge
b
AQP5
DIC
Merge
c
AQP5
DIC
Merge
d
AQP5
DIC
Merge
3

branes to the apical membranes [18, 19]. Sweating is also primarily regulated by acetylcholine, which causes an increase in intracellular calcium concentration via muscarinic receptors [2]. We therefore tried to determine whether hAQP5 translocation was regulated by an increase in intracellular calcium concentration in MDCK cells stably expressing nontagged hAQP5. Confluent monolayers of the hAQP5-MDCK cells were treated with or without (control) 10 μM of calcium ionophore A23187 for 5 or 30 min and were then subjected to an immunofluorescent analysis and a cell-side-specific biotinylation assay. In both analyses, the amount of hAQP5 protein in the apical membrane fraction increased after 5 min of A23187 treatment compared to control cells (fig. 5a, e), and it returned to the control level 30 min after this treatment (fig. 5b, f). On the other hand, the amount of hAQP5 protein in the basolateral membrane fraction did not change at either 5 or 30 min after treatment (fig. 5c, d, g, h). These results suggest that hAQP5 protein translocated relatively rapidly from the cytoplasm to the apical membranes due to an increase in intracellular calcium concentration.

Although it has been speculated that fluid moves from the interstitium to the lumen with the chloride and the sodium movements in the Na^+-K^+-$2Cl^-$ cotransport model [22], the route of the water has yet to be determined. These data showing clear immunolocalization of AQP5 in human sweat gland and translocation of AQP5 in mouse sweat gland offer new insights into the mechanism by which primary sweat is produced.

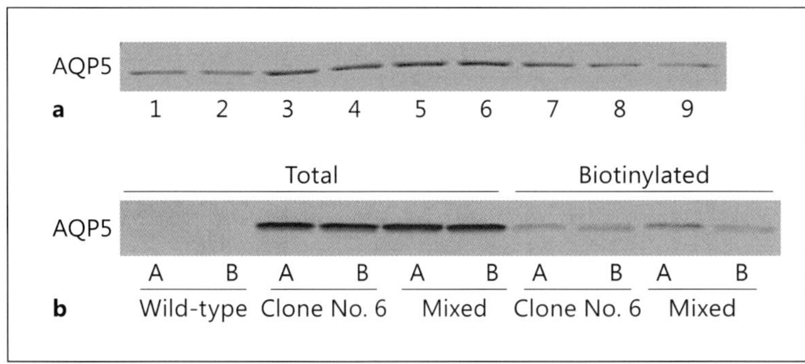

Fig. 4. Analysis of MDCK cell lines stably expressing nontagged hAQP5. **a** Nine independent clones were isolated and their expression of hAQP5 was analyzed by Western blotting. Clone No. 6, which showed a high level of AQP5 expression, and a mixture of clones Nos. 4, 7, and 9, which was used to avoid the effect of clonal variation, were selected for further experiments. **b** Localization of hAQP5 in the stable cell lines was determined by a cell-side-specific biotinylation assay. hAQP5 was detected at both the apical and basolateral sides of polarized hAQP5-MDCK cells. A = Apical membrane fraction. B = Basolateral membrane fraction. Wild-type = Wild-type MDCK cell line; mixed = mixed clone of Nos. 4, 7, and 9.

Fig. 5. hAQP5 translocation from the cytoplasm to the apical membranes of MDCK cells. **a–d** Confluent monolayers of the hAQP5-MDCK cells were treated with or without (control) 10 μM of calcium ionophore A23187, and then subjected to a cell-side-specific biotinylation assay. The figures are representative results using clone No. 6. **e–h** Densitometric analysis of **a–d** and the results using mixed clones. After 5 min of the treatment (**a**, **e**), the apical hAQP5 level increased by about twofold in A23187-treated cells, and after 30 min of the treatment (**b**, **f**) it returned to the control level. The basolateral hAQP5 level did not change after 5 or 30 min of the treatment (**c**, **d**, **g**, **h**). White bars: clone No. 6 (n = 5); black bars: mixed clone (n = 5). Error bars indicate SD. * $p < 0.05$. n.s. = Not significant.

(For figure see next page.)

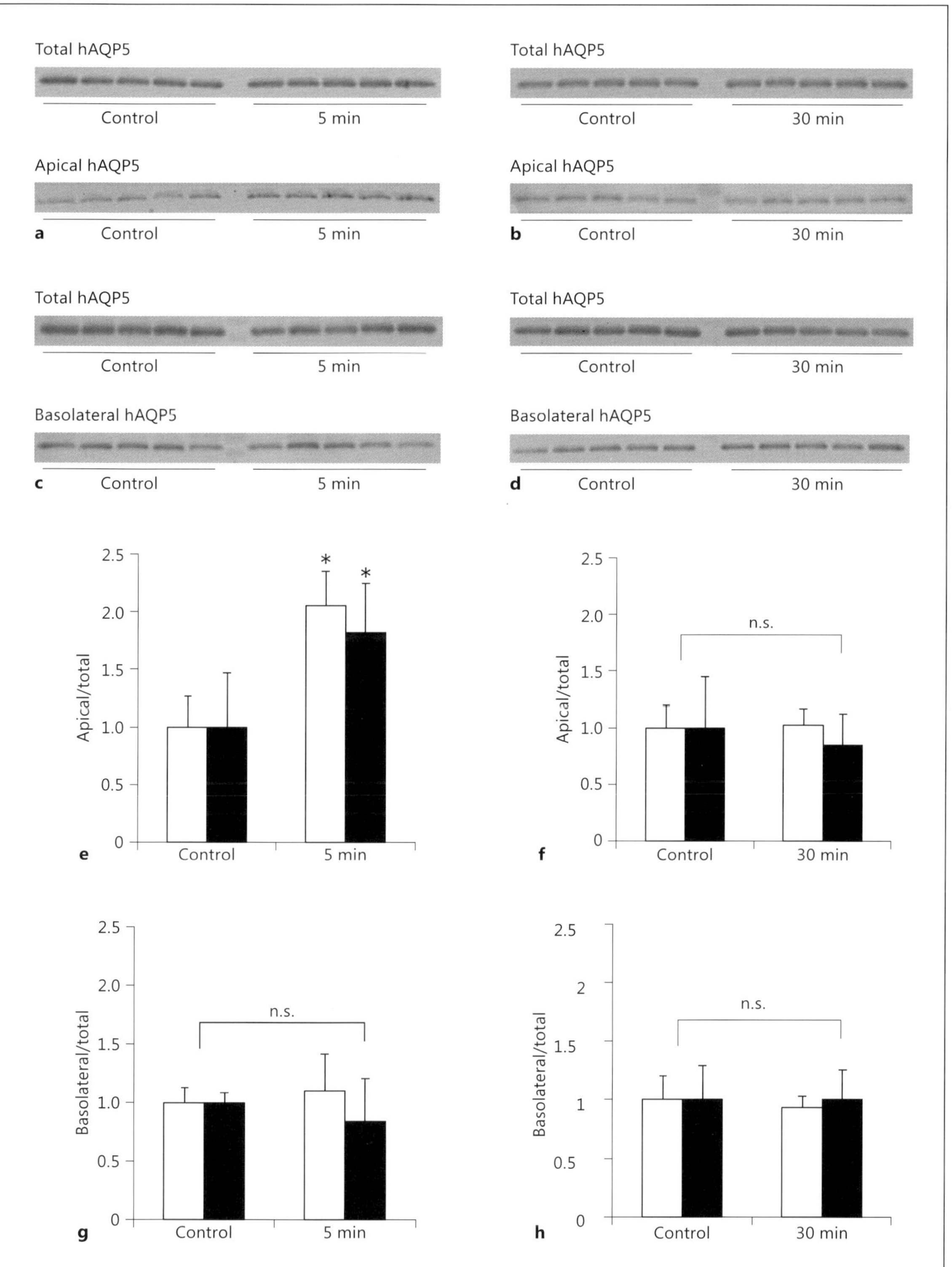
Total hAQP5
Control
5 min
Apical hAQP5
a
Control
5 min
Total hAQP5
Control
30 min
Apical hAQP5
b
Control
30 min
Total hAQP5
Control
5 min
Basolateral hAQP5
c
Control
5 min
Total hAQP5
Control
30 min
Basolateral hAQP5
d
Control
30 min
Apical/total
2.5
2.0
1.5
1.0
0.5
0
*
*
e
Control
5 min
Apical/total
n.s.
f
Control
30 min
Basolateral/total
n.s.
g
Control
5 min
Basolateral/total
2.5
2
1.5
1
0.5
0
n.s.
h
Control
30 min

5

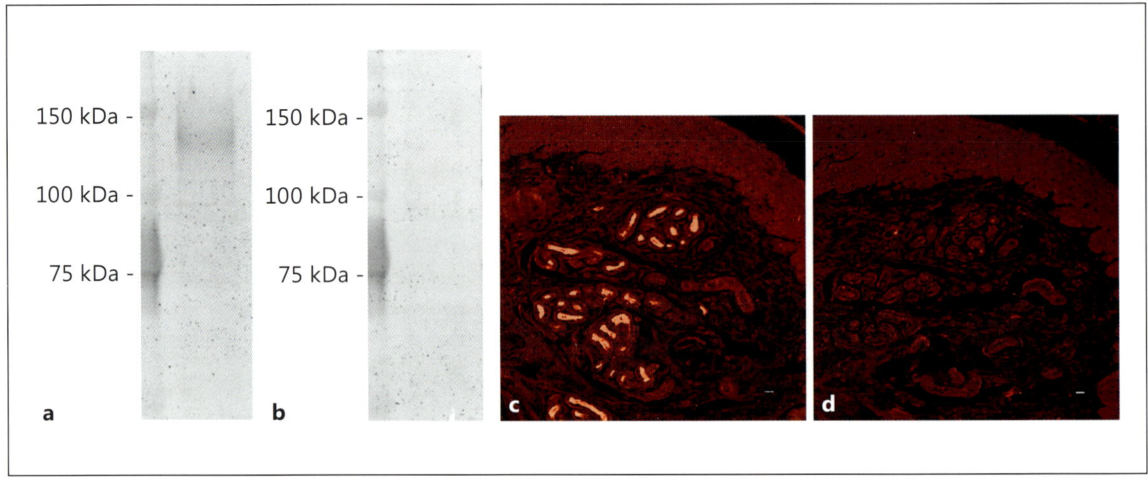

Fig. 6. ANO1 expression and localization in mouse sweat glands. **a** The anti-ANO1 antibody detected a broad band at a molecular weight of approximately 130 kDa in the immunoblot of mouse paws extract. **b** The broad band was abolished in the antibody absorption test. **c** ANO1 immunofluorescence was detected in the apical membranes of the secretory cells in a mouse sweat gland. **d** It was abolished in the antibody absorption test. Bar = 10 μm.

Anoctamin-1 Is Detected in the Apical Membranes and Colocalizes with Aquaporin-5

In addition, direct evidence for the presence of apical chloride conductance has also been lacking in the Na^+-K^+-$2Cl^-$ cotransport model. Anoctamin-1 (ANO1) is the first member of a family of calcium-activated chloride channels that were identified as anoctamins [23–25], and it has been reported to be expressed in secretory epithelial tissues where it has been implicated to play a key role in calcium-dependent chloride secretion. We thought this calcium-activated chloride channel might exist in sweat gland, so we raised the antibody to ANO1 (using the antigen peptide NH_2-C+GDGSPVPSYEYHGDAL-COOH, corresponding to amino acid residues 941–956 of mouse ANO1) and investigated ANO1 protein expression and localization in mouse sweat glands. The anti-ANO1 antibody detected a broad band at a molecular weight of approximately 130 kDa in the immunoblot of the mouse paws extract (fig. 6a), and ANO1 immunofluorescence was detected in the apical membranes of the secretory cells in a mouse sweat gland (fig. 6c).

We then performed double-immunofluorescent analysis of ANO1 and AQP5 (sc-9890) in histological sections of the mice paws under nonsweating and sweating conditions. ANO1 was detected only in the apical membranes under both conditions, and it completely colocalized with AQP5 in these apical membranes (fig. 7). In contrast to AQP5, the localization of ANO1 did not differ under the different applied conditions. With the data that ANO1 does not need trafficking regulation, it made sense to us that AQP5 apical translocation is not a general characteristic of apical membrane proteins involved in sweating. We consider ANO1 to only be the chloride channel in the apical membranes in the Na^+-K^+-$2Cl^-$ cotransport model, or at least is one type of the chloride channels for which the direct evidence of the histochemical localization have been lacking.

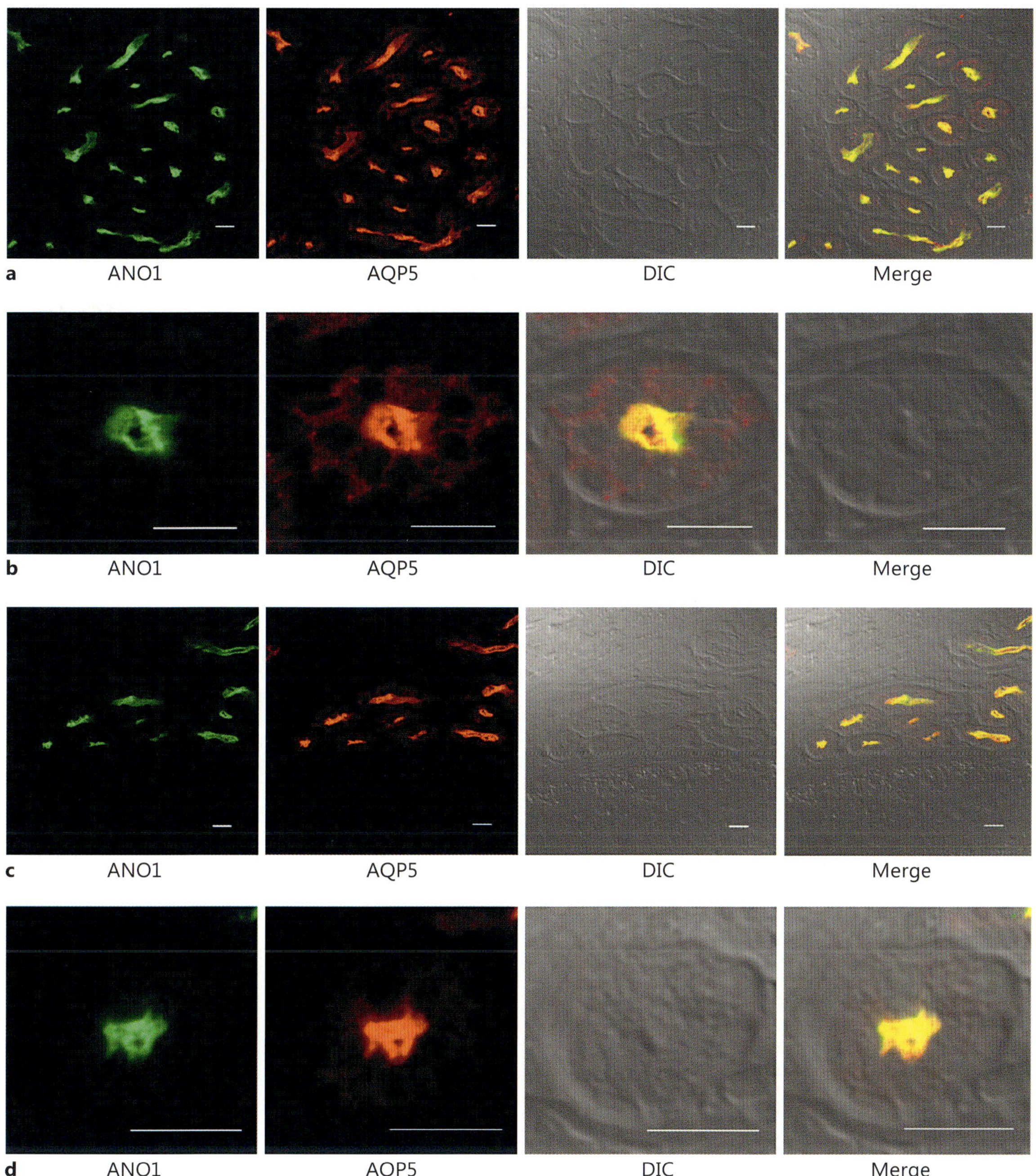

Fig. 7. Colocalization of ANO1 and AQP5 in mouse sweat glands. Double-immunofluorescent staining of ANO1 (green) and AQP5 (red) in histological sections of the paw of a representative mouse under nonsweating or sweating conditions are shown. **a**, **b** Under nonsweating condition, immunoreactive ANO1 was detected in the apical membranes of the secretory cells and partially colocalized with AQP5. **c**, **d** Under sweating condition, immunoreactive ANO1 was detected in the apical membranes of these cells and colocalized with AQP5 in the apical membranes. The cellular localization of ANO1 did not change during sweating. Bar = 10 μm. DIC = Differential interference contrast.

Aquaporin-5 in Sweat Glands

Regarding the role of AQP5 in sweat glands, the previous knockout mouse studies reported contradictory results: one study demonstrated dramatically reduced sweating in AQP5 null ($^{-/-}$) mice [7], while the other study demonstrated no significant difference in sweating between wild-type mice and AQP5 null ($^{-/-}$) mice [6]. The reason for this discrepancy is not clear at present, but our study clearly showed the existence of regulated apical translocation of AQP5 in sweat glands, which may contribute to sweat secretion by increasing the water permeability of the apical plasma membranes of sweat glands.

The findings of our study provide new insights into the mechanism by which primary sweat is produced. Agents that modulate AQP5 function or ANO1 function may be useful for the treatment of patients with sweating disorders. Further investigation is required.

References

1 Dobson RL, Sato K: The secretion of salt and water by the eccrine sweat gland. Arch Dermatol 1972;105:366–370.

2 Sato K: The physiology, pharmacology, and biochemistry of the eccrine sweat gland. Rev Physiol Biochem Pharmacol 1977;79:51–131.

3 Ishibashi K, Hara S, Kondo S: Aquaporin water channels in mammals. Clin Exp Nephrol 2009;13:107–117.

4 Ma L, Huang YG, He H, Deng YC, Zhang HF, Che HL, Tian JY, Zhao G: Postnatal expression and denervation induced up-regulation of aquaporin-5 protein in rat sweat gland. Cell Tissue Res 2007; 329:25–33.

5 Ma L, Huang YG, Deng YC, Tian JY, Rao ZR, Che HL, Zhang HF, Zhao G: Topiramate reduced sweat secretion and aquaporin-5 expression in sweat glands of mice. Life Sci 2007;80:2461–2468.

6 Song Y, Sonawane N, Verkman AS: Localization of aquaporin-5 in sweat glands and functional analysis using knockout mice. J Physiol 2002;541:561–568.

7 Nejsum LN, Kwon TH, Jensen UB, Fumagalli O, Frøkiaer J, Krane CM, Menon AG, King LS, Agre PC, Nielsen S: Functional requirement of aquaporin-5 in plasma membranes of sweat glands. Proc Natl Acad Sci USA 2002;99:511–516.

8 Iizuka T, Suzuki T, Nakano K, Sueki H: Immunolocalization of aquaporin 5 in normal human skin and hypohidrotic skin diseases. J Dermatol 2012;39:344–349.

9 Kabashima K, Shimauchi T, Kobayashi M, Fukamachi S, Kawakami C, Ogata M, Kabashima R, Mori T, Ota T, Fukushima S, Hara-Chikuma M, Tokura Y: Aberrant aquaporin 5 expression in the sweat gland in aquagenic wrinkling of the palms. J Am Acad Dermatol 2008; 59:S28–S32.

10 Inoue R, Sohara E, Rai T, Satoh T, Yokozeki H, Sasaki S, Uchida S: Immunolocalization and translocation of aquaporin-5 water channel in sweat glands. J Dermatol Sci 2013;70:26–33.

11 Quinton PM, Tormey JM: Localization of Na/K-ATPase sites in the secretory and reabsorptive epithelia of perfused eccrine sweat glands: a question to the role of the enzyme in secretion. J Membr Biol 1976;29:383–399.

12 Saga K, Sato K: Ultrastructural localization of ouabain-sensitive, K-dependent p-nitrophenyl phosphatase activity in monkey eccrine sweat gland. J Histochem Cytochem 1988;36:1023–1030.

13 Zhang M, Zeng S, Zhang L, Li H, Chen L, Zhang X, Li X, Lin C, Shu S, Xie S, He Y, Mao X, Peng L, Shi L, Yang L, Tang S, Fu X: Localization of Na^+-K^+-ATPase α/β, Na^+-K^+-2Cl-cotransporter 1 and aquaporin-5 in human eccrine sweat glands. Acta Histochem 2014;116:1374–1381.

14 Yamamoto T, Sasaki S, Fushimi K, Ishibashi K, Yaoita E, Kawasaki K, Marumo F, Kihara I: Vasopressin increases AQP CD water channel in apical membrane of collecting duct cells in Brattleboro rats. Am J Physiol 1995;268:C1546–C1551.

15 Nielsen S, DiGiovanni SR, Christensen EI, Knepper MA, Harris HW: Cellular and subcellular immunolocalization of vasopressin-regulated water channel in rat kidney. Proc Natl Acad Sci USA 1993;90:11663–11667.

16 Fushimi K, Uchida S, Hara Y, Hirata Y, Marumo F, Sasaki S: Cloning and expression of apical membrane water channel of rat kidney collecting tubule. Nature 1993;361:549–552.

17 Raina S, Preston GM, Guggino WB, Agre P: Molecular cloning and characterization of an aquaporin cDNA from salivary, lacrimal, and respiratory tissues. J Biol Chem 1995;270:1908–1912.

18 Ishikawa Y, Eguchi T, Skowronski MT, Ishida H: Acetylcholine acts on M_3 muscarinic receptors and induces the translocation of aquaporin5 water channel via cytosolic $Ca2^+$ elevation in rat parotid glands. Biochem Biophys Res Commun 1998;245:835–840.

19 Ishikawa Y, Skowronski MT, Inoue N, Ishida H: α_1-Adrenoceptor-induced trafficking of aquaporin-5 to the apical plasma membrane of rat parotid cells. Biochem Biophys Res Commun 1999;265: 94–100.

20 Ishikawa Y, Yuan Z, Inoue N, Skowronski MT, Nakae Y, Shono M, Cho G, Yasui M, Agre P, Nielsen S: Identification of AQP5 in lipid rafts and its translocation to apical membranes by activation of M_3 mAChRs in interlobular ducts of rat parotid gland. Am J Physiol Cell Physiol 2005;289:C1303–C1311.

21 Kosugi-Tanaka C, Li X, Yao C, Akamatsu T, Kanamori N, Hosoi K: Protein kinase A-regulated membrane trafficking of a green fluorescent protein-aquaporin 5 chimera in MDCK cells. Biochim Biophys Acta 2006;1763:337–344.
22 Saga K: Structure and function of human sweat glands studied with histochemistry and cytochemistry. Prog Histochem Cytochem 2002;37:323–386.
23 Caputo A, Caci E, Ferrera L, Pedemonte N, Barsanti C, Sondo E, Pfeffer U, Ravazzolo R, Zegarra-Moran O, Galietta LJ: TMEM16A, a membrane protein associated with calcium-dependent chloride channel activity. Science 2008;322:590–594.
24 Yang YD, Cho H, Koo JY, Tak MH, Cho Y, Shim WS, Park SP, Lee J, Lee B, Kim BM, Raouf R, Shin YK, Oh U: TMEM16A confers receptor-activated calcium-dependent chloride conductance. Nature 2008;455:1210–1215.
25 Schroeder BC, Cheng T, Jan YN, Jan LY: Expression cloning of TMEM16A as a calcium-activated chloride channel subunit. Cell 2008;134:1019–1029.

Risako Inoue, MD, PhD
Department of Dermatology
Graduate School of Medical and Dental Sciences
Tokyo Medical and Dental University
1-5-45 Yushima, Bunkyo-ku
Tokyo 113-8510 (Japan)
E-Mail risa_derm@yahoo.co.jp

Yokozeki H, Murota H, Katayama I (eds): Perspiration Research.
Curr Probl Dermatol. Basel, Karger, 2016, vol 51, pp 22–29 (DOI: 10.1159/000446755)

Old and New Approaches for Assessing Sweating

Hiroyuki Murota

Department of Dermatology, Course of Integrated Medicine, Graduate School of Medicine, Osaka University, Osaka, Japan

Abstract

The evaluation of sweating activities contributes to both medical services and social living. There are several old and new approaches for assessing sweating. These methods are mainly composed of adopted techniques that focus on detecting small amounts of water on the skin surface. For many years, the iodine-starch reaction has been applied in various settings to evaluate sweat on the skin surface. However, methodology based on the coloration of sweat is in a constant state of evolution, and multiple advancements have been made. Furthermore, common fingerprinting is not just used for obtaining personal-identifying information anymore as it can also provide scientifically important information for sweat-pore mapping and sweat-component analysis. Additionally, there are multiple techniques for the quantitative measurement of sweat volume and dynamic intravital imaging of sweat, and these are also continually evolving. This chapter provides an overview of the old and new approaches for assessing sweating.

Coloration of Sweat

Minor Method and Iodine-Starch Reaction-Related Methods

The presence of sweat on the skin surface is often confirmed by the iodine-starch reaction [1], which is based on the fact that water from sweat dyes starch in the presence of iodine. Historically, the original Minor method used a tincture of iodine, whereas the improved method utilizes a compound liquid containing iodine (3 g), castor oil (20 g), and ethanol (200 ml) [2]. Briefly, affected regions of skin are evenly painted with iodine solution, and starch powder is sprinkled on top after it dries. Based on the assay sensitivity, this method is suitable for evaluating moderate-to-heavy sweating and has been used to assess thermal sweating from both whole-body and segmented/localized hyperhidrosis.

To date, numerous modifications have been incorporated to improve the assay sensitivity of the Minor method. Sato et al. [3], for example, devised the one-step iodine-starch method. In preparation for this procedure, a solution containing soluble starch mixed with iodine (500 and 5 g, respectively) is prepared and sealed for approximately 1 week. At the examination, the yellowish (by sublimation of iodine) soluble starch is evenly sprinkled onto the skin surface and dyed by sweat. The advantages of this method are: (1) higher assay sensitivity compared to the Minor method, (2) a one-step straightforward procedure, and (3) decreased harmfulness due to elimination of other test reagents. A disadvantage of this method, however, is the difficulty involved in sprinkling the soluble starch powder evenly on a curved surface. That is, when we put this powder on the curved surface of dry skin, it falls off. Thus, this method requires some ingenuity, such as covering the powdered skin in wrapping film.

Wada [4] reported another improved method with a higher degree of sensitivity for using the iodine-starch reaction to detect sweat. In this assay, a tincture of ~2–3% iodine is first applied evenly to the skin, followed by painting of the region with a mixed suspension of starch-castor oil (50–100 and 100 g, respectively). This modification provides increased sensitivity for the detection of sweat (fig. 1).

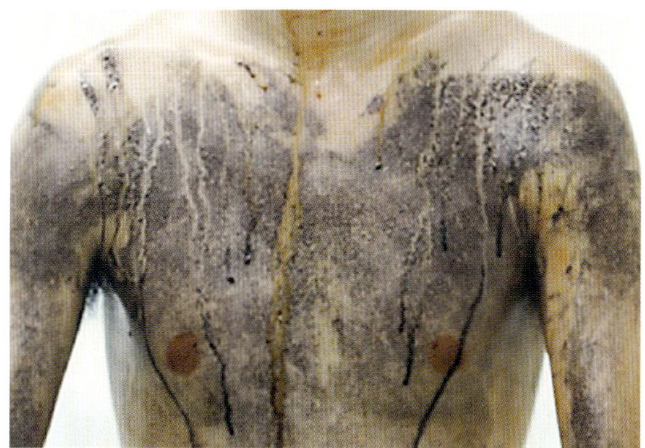

Fig. 1. Visualization of the sweat response in a healthy volunteer using the iodine-starch method of Wada.

Colored Sweat Drop Replicas

The most familiar way to obtain a sweat drop replica is via the iodine paper method. This methodology has successively been improved upon by Yokozeki et al. [1]. In their modified procedure, hot air-dried photocopying paper (100 g) is kept in a sealed desiccator with iodine (1 g) for about 1 week [1]. The yellowish photocopying paper, referred to as iodine paper, can bear long-term storage. During examination, the skin to be tested is put into direct contact with the iodine paper. The duration of contact can be up to several dozen seconds and is adjusted according to sweat volume. The sweat drop replicas will appear as a dyeing of the iodine paper. Importantly, the test results as they appear on the iodine paper are not permanent. Therefore, to preserve those findings, it is necessary to make a copy or photo of the dyed paper.

The direct staining of pores containing sweat is a promising way to investigate the distribution of active sweat glands. In the iodine-Formvar method, the skin is painted with a 5% tincture of iodine, and subsequently, a mixed solution of Formvar (polyvinyl formal) (0.5 g), ethylene dischloride containing 3% butyl phthalate (10 ml), and starch (4 g) is applied. The film that forms on the skin surface contains sweat drops, which appear as black-purple spots. This provides a map of active sweat pores and can be stored for long periods of time [1]. *o*-Phthalaldehyde is also used to stain active sweat pores based on its unique characteristic of becoming discolored in response to ammonia [5]. The stain solution is prepared by solubilizing *o*-phthalaldehyde (5%) in xylene or ethyl ether, and this is applied directly on the skin. After a few minutes, the pores with sweat will be stained black in color.

Other Methods for Obtaining Replicas of Sweat Drops and Sweat Pores

Silicon rubber can be used to investigate the anatomical localization of active sweat pores [6]. Ordinarily, unset medical silicon rubber, which is often used to make models of teeth, is placed on the skin and allowed to set. During this process, sweat from sweat pores will push up the unset silicon gum and will make replicas on the silicon layer. The set silicon rubber also provides a record of the skin surface texture. Thus, although it is less quantitative than other methods, silicon rubber is useful for understanding the anatomical location of active sweat pores.

Fingerprinting can also provide important information, not only for individual discrimination, but also for sweat-pore mapping and sweat-component analysis. Lee et al. [7] focused on the unique function of hydrochromic polymers (polydiacetylenes), a water-responsive sensor that undergoes a blue-to-red color transition. Polydiacetylenes can detect tiny amounts of water on skin surface and utilize them in 'hydrochromic mapping of human sweat pores'. This mapping method is also useful for distinguishing active and inactive sweat glands. Recently, in order to connect information from high-resolution fingerprint scans with chemical information from sweat, Elsner and Abel [8] described the utility of a thin film of gold to obtain a complete fingerprint with the exact positions of sweat pores. These strategies are expected to expand the availability of fingerprinting for the application of public, forensic, and medical sciences.

Measurement of Sweat Volume

Gravimetric Method
Sweat volume is frequently determined by the gravimetric method, which involves measuring the weight of sweat soaked into filter paper. In this assay, to avoid the influences of environmental humidity, an airtight space should be prepared on the surface of skin to be tested. It is also recommended that the filter paper used in this assay is either an ash-less grade or is presoaked with 0.25% acetic acid and dried. Briefly, the weight of the filter paper is measured, and it is then put in the airtight space on the skin to collect sweat. The paper is then weighed again, and the difference in weight of filter paper before versus after collection indicates the sweat volume. When determining the weight of the filter paper, it is important that this paper be set in a sealed vial to avoid the influence of environmental humidity [1].

Collection of Sweat
Anaerobic Method. To evaluate the sweat volume from a broader area of the body, the modified anaerobic method of sweat collection, reported by Boysen et al. [9] and Yokozeki et al. [1], is useful. In this assay, a broad area of the body is covered by a vinyl bag, which is then sealed with tape. Of note, the skin to be tested should be applied with petroleum jelly (e.g. Vaseline) topically in advance. Sweat will run off the surface of the petroleum jelly and will be less contaminated by substances on the skin surface. The volume of collected sweat in the vinyl bag can then be measured. This method is also useful for collecting sweat for subsequent biochemical component analysis.
Yokozeki's Method. In contrast to the anaerobic method, which collects sweat from a broad area of the body, the modified method of Yokozeki et al. [10] is designed to collect sweat from a smaller area in the center of the back. Briefly, the whole back is wiped with saline and draped with an opened square measuring 40 × 50 cm, followed by applying Vaseline on the back. Subjects enter a sauna (80 °C) and under aerobic conditions the pooled sweat in the draped cloth square is collected with a syringe. As it is assumed that components of sweat will vary considerably with loca-

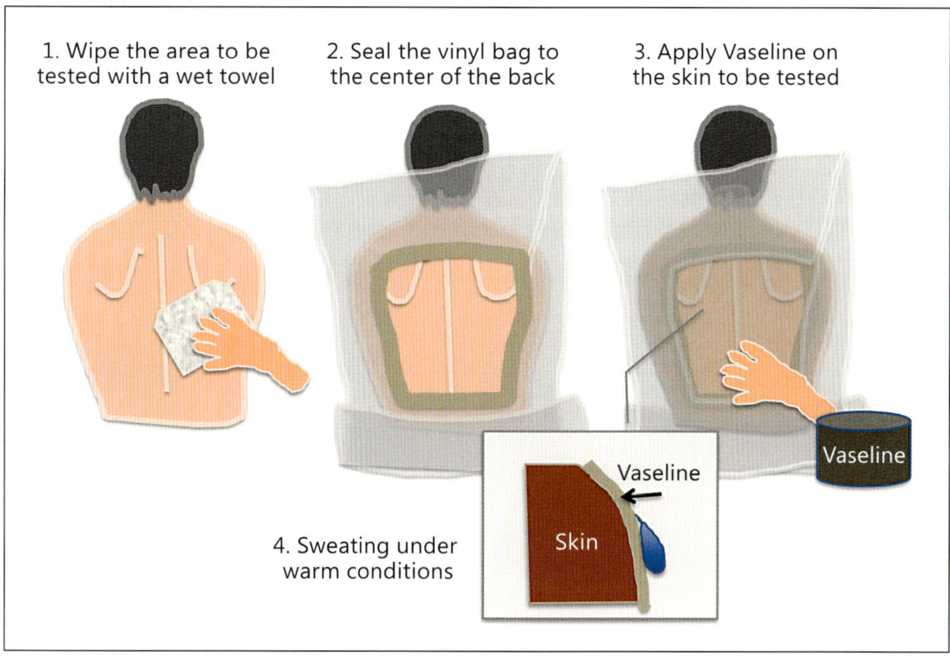

Fig. 2. Illustration of the Yokozeki sweat collection method.

tion, this method has the advantage of obtaining fairly uniform sweat (fig. 2).

Ventilated Capsule Technique

Basic. The basic ventilated capsule technique quantitatively measures the volume of water evaporating from the skin surface by attaching a ventilation capsule directly onto the skin surface [11]. Based on the traditional measuring principle, the humidity of both the dry air, which is sent into the capsule, and the moist air that is extruded out from capsule, is measured. The difference in humidity is then recorded as the sweat volume. This technique enables the quantitative real-time measurement of temporal changes in sweat volume.

Application: Quantitative Sudomotor Axon Reflex Testing. The ventilated capsule technique can be applied for the quantitative measurement of the volume of axon reflex-mediated sweating [12, 13]. In this assay, a ventilated sweat capsule is attached with an additional outward sponge compartment, which assumes the role of iontophoresis (fig. 3). From the outward compartment, acetylcholine (approx. 100 mg/ml) is iontophoretically applied to skin, and this will induce sweat via activation of the axon reflex. Quantitative sudomotor axon reflex testing can provide the axon reflex-mediated sweat volume, as well as the latency time to sweat. If the volume is low and/or the latency time is prolonged, this suggests a postganglionic sympathetic abnormality or an abnormality in the microenvironment surrounding the sweat gland.

Skin Conductance

Skin hydration is often evaluated by the conductance method, which is based on the fact that sweat will moisten the skin surface. Moistened skin develops an increase in electrical conductiv-

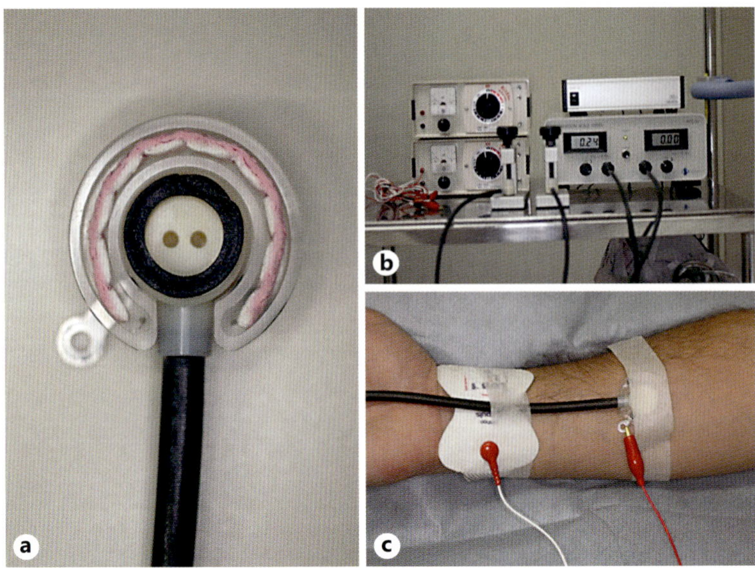

Fig. 3. Devices for quantitative sudomotor axon reflex testing. **a** A ventilation sweat capsule attached to an outer cavity for acetylcholine iontophoresis. **b** Instruments for quantitative sudomotor axon reflex testing: the electric power source for iontophoresis is on the left, and the device for measurement of sweat is on the right. **c** The ventilation sweat capsule should be attached to the surface of skin. Reprinted from Kijima et al. [13] with permission of the Japanese Society of Allergology.

ity. An electric conductivity apparatus can measure the electric conductance of skin by putting a probe on the surface. The usefulness of this method was first proven in mice, which have functional sweat glands in their foot paws but not in the back skin. Accordingly, skin hydration will significantly increase on acetylcholine-treated foot paws, but not on acetylcholine-treated back skin, which has no sweat glands, and the difference in skin conductance between the two regions is reflective of sweat volume [14]. It should be noted that skin hydration will be influenced by the environmental humidity and the situation at the time of examination.

Sympathetic Skin Response

The sympathetic skin response has been used in the evaluation of sweat gland activity, and involves measuring the electric potential of skin after sudomotor treatment, such as with electric stimulation [15]. The change in the electric potential before versus after treatment can be regarded as sweat gland activity. Sudomotor treatment develops a sodium concentration gradient inside the sweat glands. Due to sodium reabsorption from the sweat duct, the sodium concentration of fresh sweat in the gland is high, whereas the amount of sodium in sweat near the skin surface is low. This change in the concentration gradient develops an electrical potential. Although this method is useful for understanding the autonomic function with little effort, the result is only semiquantitative. To overcome this issue, the sympathetic sweat response method quantitatively measures the sweat volume on palms and soles induced by sudomotor treatment by using a ventilation sweat capsule [16].

Dynamic Imaging of Sweat and Sweat Glands

Optical Coherence Tomography
Optical coherence tomography (OCT) is a noninvasive imaging technology that can obtain both the cross-sectional and 3-dimensional image of a tissue using light. During examination with OCT,

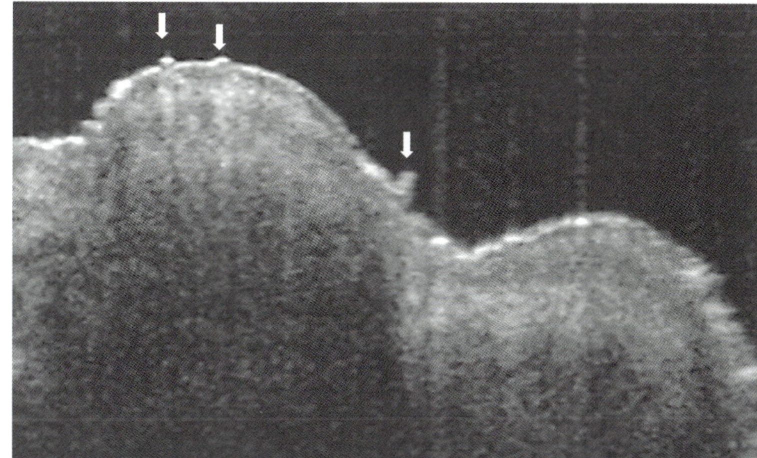

Fig. 4. Observation of intravital sweat movement by OCT. Arrows indicates sweat. This image was created from a collaboration with Professor Masato Ohmi, Biomedical Optics Laboratory, Division of Health Sciences, Osaka University.

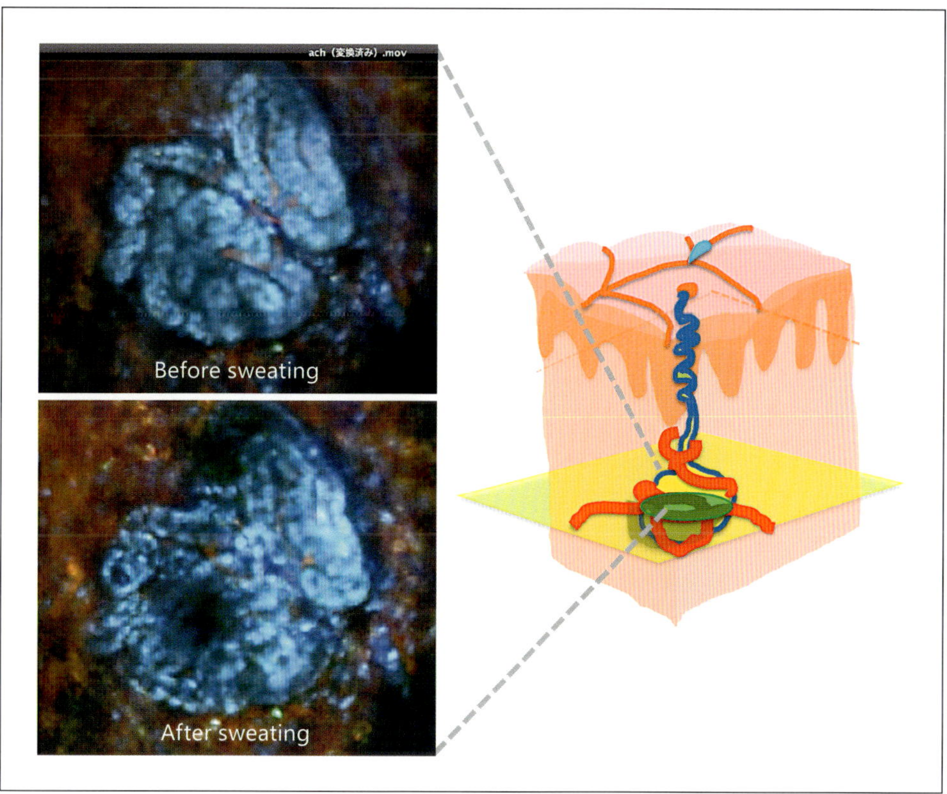

Fig. 5. Visualization of intravital sweat gland movement by 2-photon microscopic analysis. Green: sweat glands detected by the AQP5 antibody conjugated with FITC. Red: blood vessels stained with dextran conjugated with Texas Red. Blue: nuclear staining with Hoechst. The opaque spot observed after sweating indicates sweat. This image was created from a collaboration with Professor Masaru Ishii and Professor Junichi Kikuta, Department of Immunology and Cell Biology, Graduate School of Medicine and Frontier Biosciences, Osaka University.

water appears as a strong signal by white-light interferometry [17]. Thus, movement of sweat inside the stratum corneum and the epidermis can be observed up to a depth of 100 μm. Furthermore, because there is a large refractive index difference on the wall of the spiral lumen between the sweat and the keratinous epidermal tissues, the eccrine sweat ducts in the stratum corneum of the epidermis are clearly recognized by a high reflective light intensity. Thus, the dynamic OCT images of sweating in the x-z plane can be obtained (fig. 4). A limitation of this method, however, is the observable depth, and at present it is difficult to make a direct observation of sweat glands by OCT.

OSM

Two-Photon Excitation Fluorescence Microscopy
To obtain both structural and functional information about sweat glands, intravital multiphoton imaging of these glands in murine paws has been performed using previously described protocols [18], with some modifications [14]. Briefly, mice are anesthetized with isoflurane, and their paws are observed with an inverted multiphoton microscope driven by a Ti:Sapphire laser tuned to 800 nm and an inverted microscope equipped with multi-immersion objectives. Sweat glands can be visualized by antimuscarinic receptor 3 or antiaquaporin 5 (AQP5) antibody staining. Simultaneously visualizing blood vessels with Texas Red-labeled 70-kDa dextran and performing nuclear staining can also be helpful for understanding the tissue orientation. Images of sweat gland activity obtained via this method are shown in figure 5, online supplementary video 1 (see www.karger.com/doi/10.1159/000446755 for all online suppl. material), and online supplementary video 2. Sweat glands were stained green using the AQP5 antibody conjugated with fluorescein isothiocyanate (FITC), and the capillary vessels were visualized by dextran conjugated with Texas Red; cell nuclei are in blue. After acetylcholine administration, the sweat gland writhes, followed by the appearance of opaque spots (fig. 5). It can reasonably be assumed that these spots are derived from the change in local pH, i.e. acidification due to sweating [14].

References

1 Yokozeki H, et al: Assessment of sweating; in Nishiyama S, Nishikawa T, Nishioka K (eds): Handbook for Dermatological Laboratory Procedure, ed 1. Tokyo, Nankodo, 1991 (in Japanese).
2 Minor V: Ein neues Verfahren zu der klinischen Untersuchung der Schweissabsonderung. Dtsch Z Nervenheilkd 1928, pp 101302–101307.
3 Sato KT, et al: One-step iodine method for direct visualization of sweating. Am J Med Sci 1988;295;528–531.
4 Wada M: Sudorific action of adrenaline on the human sweat glands and determination of their excitability. Science 1950;111;376–377.
5 Ohman S, Shelley WB: *o*-Phthalaldehyde staining of coiled and uncoiled intraepidermal sweat ducts. J Invest Dermatol 1969;53:29–33.
6 Sarkany I, Gaylarde PM: A silicon rubber technique to demonstrate sweat gland activity. J Invest Dermatol 1972; 59:269.
7 Lee J, et al: Hydrochromic conjugated polymers for human sweat pore mapping. Nat Commun 2014;5:3736.
8 Elsner C, Abel B: Ultrafast high-resolution mass spectrometric finger pore imaging in latent finger prints. Sci Rep 2014;4:6905.
9 Boysen TC, Yanagawa S, Sato F, Sato K: A modified anaerobic method of sweat collection. J Appl Physiol Respir Environ Exerc Physiol 1984;56:1302–1307.
10 Yokozeki H, Hibino T, Takemura T, Sato K: Cysteine proteinase inhibitor in eccrine sweat is derived from sweat gland. Am J Physiol 1991;260:R314–R320.
11 McLean JA: Measurement of cutaneous moisture vaporization from cattle by ventilated capsules. J Physiol 1963;167: 417–426.
12 Lee JB: Heat acclimatization in hot summer for ten weeks suppress the sensitivity of sweating in response to iontophoretically-administered acetylcholine. Korean J Physiol Pharmacol 2008;12: 349–355.
13 Kijima A, Murota H, Matsui S, Takahashi A, Kimura A, Kitaba S, Lee JB, Katayama I: Abnormal axon reflex-mediated sweating correlates with high state of anxiety in atopic dermatitis. Allergol Int 2012;61:469–473.

14 Matsui S, Murota H, Takahashi A, Yang L, Lee JB, Omiya K, Ohmi M, Kikuta J, Ishii M, Katayama I: Dynamic analysis of histamine-mediated attenuation of acetylcholine-induced sweating via GSK3β activation. J Invest Dermatol 2014;134:326–334.
15 Baser SM, Meer J, Polinsky RJ, Hallett M: Sudomotor function in autonomic failure. Neurology 1991;41:1564–1566.
16 Asahina M, Kikkawa Y, Suzuki A, Hattori T: Cutaneous sympathetic function in patients with multiple system atrophy. Clin Auton Res 2003;13:91–95.
17 Ohmi M, Tanigawa M, Yamada A, Ueda Y, Haruna M: Dynamic analysis of internal and external mental sweating by optical coherence tomography. J Biomed Opt 2009;14:014026.
18 Ishii M, Egen JG, Klauschen F, Meier-Schellersheim M, Saeki Y, Vacher J, Proia RL, Germain RN: Sphingosine-1-phosphate mobilizes osteoclast precursors and regulates bone homeostasis. Nature 2009;458:524–528.

Hiroyuki Murota
Department of Dermatology
Course of Integrated Medicine
Graduate School of Medicine
Osaka University
2-2 Yamadaoka, Suita-shi
Osaka 565-0871 (Japan)
E-Mail h-murota@derma.med.osaka-u.ac.jp

Yokozeki H, Murota H, Katayama I (eds): Perspiration Research.
Curr Probl Dermatol. Basel, Karger, 2016, vol 51, pp 30–41 (DOI: 10.1159/000446756)

Sweat as an Efficient Natural Moisturizer

Tetsuo Shiohara · Yohei Sato · Yurie Komatsu · Yukiko Ushigome · Yoshiko Mizukawa

Department of Dermatology, Kyorin University School of Medicine, Tokyo, Japan

Abstract

Although recent research on the pathogenesis of allergic skin diseases such as atopic dermatitis has focused on defects in skin genes important for maintaining skin barrier function, the fact that excreted sweat has an overwhelmingly great capacity to increase skin surface hydration and contains moisturizing factors has long been ignored: the increase in water loss induced by these gene defects could theoretically be compensated fully by a significant increase in sweating. In this review, the dogma postulating the detrimental role of sweat in these diseases has been challenged on the basis of recent findings on the physiological functions of sweat, newly recognized sweat gland-/duct-related skin diseases, and therapeutic approaches to the management of these diseases. We are now beginning to appreciate that sweat glands/ducts are a sophisticated regulatory system. Furthermore, depending on their anatomical location and the degree of the impairment, this system might have a different function: sweating responses in sweat glands/ducts located at the folds in hairy skin such as on the trunk and extremities could function as natural regulators that maintain skin hydration under quiescent basal conditions, in addition to the better-studied thermoregulatory functions, which can be mainly mediated by those at the ridges. The normal functioning of sweat could be disturbed in various inflammatory skin diseases. Thus, we should recognize sweating disturbance as an etiologic factor in the development of these diseases.

Sweat is generally thought to be an important factor in the exacerbation of several clinical symptoms in many allergic skin diseases [1]. Indeed, many patients with allergic skin diseases often complain of aggravation of pruritus and eczematous skin lesions after severe sweating. The prevailing dogma, which is shaped by such observations, has depicted the detrimental role of sweat in allergic inflammation. However, the role of sweat in allergic inflammation is more complex than previous studies have implied: there is increasing evidence of the protective role of sweat on allergic inflammation, such as atopic dermatitis (AD). First, AD skin lesions, particularly in adult patients, often spare well-hydrated flexural areas, such as axillae, which are also characterized by increased sweating. Second, AD patients, who characteristically have itchy skin, often experience spontaneous remission in summer, although this remission may result in part from environmental factors, such as high ambient humidity and temperature. Third, infants born in autumn show the highest prevalence of AD, while those born in spring show the lowest [2]. Fourth, dermcidin (DCD), a new antimicrobial peptide exclusively produced by eccrine sweat glands, contributes to the first line of defense against invading pathogens by building a constant barrier that overlies the epithelial skin [3]. Fifth, excreted sweat has an overwhelmingly great capacity to increase skin surface hydration (SSH) and contains moisturizing factors, such as lactate, urea, sodium, and potassium, to maintain skin hydration [4]. Thus, the maintenance of normal skin hydration is an important function of sweat.

In view of the fact that the water content of sweat is much higher than that in transepidermal water loss, the increase in water loss induced by the loss-of-function mutations in the gene encoding filaggrin *(FRG)* [5, 6] could theoretically be compensated fully by a significant increase in sweating. Research on the regulation of sweating responses under various pathophysiologic conditions, however, have been hampered by the paucity of reproducible and quantitative evaluation methods, although a variety of methods for sweat testing have been devised: there is still a need for a sensitive and specific test. In this regard, we have recently established a useful method, the impression mold technique (IMT), which allows an accurate quantification of individual sweat glands/ducts actively delivering sweat and the volume of sweat they produce over time [7] (fig. 1). This test provides an assessment of individual sweat droplet number and size in different regions, thereby making it possible to estimate individual sweat gland/duct activity to secrete sweat.

Moisturizers are widely used by many patients with allergic skin diseases to alleviate clinical symptoms by increasing skin hydration. Because excreted sweat can markedly relieve skin dryness and attenuate nonhistaminergic pruritus in the skin of AD patients [8], increasing sweating could be more efficient at maintaining skin hydration and alleviating allergic inflammation than applying moisturizers. Thus, the prevailing dogma postulating the deleterious role of sweat in allergic inflammation has been challenged by several recent findings. The aim of the present paper is to briefly review recent findings on the physiological function of sweating, newly recognized sweat gland-related diseases, and therapeutic approaches to the management of these diseases.

Physiological Functions of Sweat

In humans, eccrine sweat glands are distributed widely on both hairy and glabrous skin, such as the palms and soles, with some exceptions [9]. In contrast, other mammals, such as monkeys, dogs, and mice, have eccrine glands only on glabrous skin, such as the paw. Sweat pores of eccrine glands in hairy skin open at the skin folds (fig. 1), while those in the glabrous skin open at the dermal ridges [10]. Thus, there are substantial differences in function between sweat pores in hairy skin and glabrous skin: those located in the glabrous skin of the palms and soles secrete sweat in response to emotional or psychological stress, physical exercise, and high environmental temperatures. In contrast, those located in the hairy skin do not necessarily respond well to such stimuli [11]. Eccrine glands first appear around the 4th gestational month during embryonic development in the glabrous skin of the palms and soles and then spread to the rest of the body, such as the hairy skin, at the 5th month [12]: the emergence of eccrine glands in glabrous skin may precede that in hairy skin during evolution. This classification, however, is too simplified because even in the hairy skin, sweat pores open not only at the skin folds but also at the ridges.

To investigate whether the function of sweat would be different depending on the localization

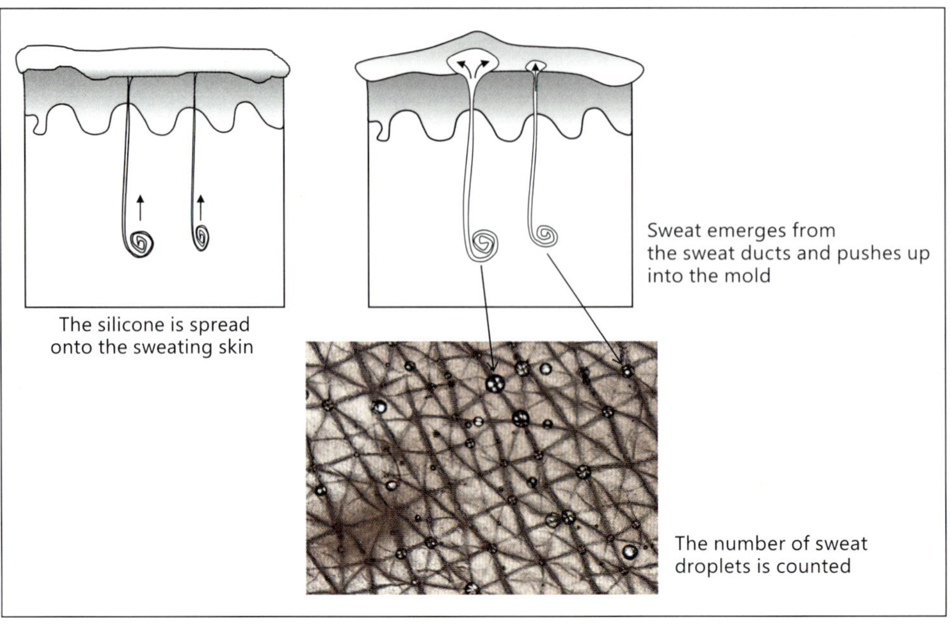

Fig. 1. IMT for the assessment of sweating responses. The silicone material is mixed with a water solution and spread onto the skin. As the silicone hardens, it retains the impression of the sweat droplets as they emerge from the sweat ducts and push up into the mold. Impression molds harden in 3–4 min and then they are removed. The resulting sweat droplets are counted using a dissecting microscope and quantified by number and size per area over a 1-cm^2 region. Sweat droplets usually occupy each dermal fold in the hairy skin and are rarely detected in the ridges in healthy subjects before thermal stimulus.

of sweat pores relative to skin folds and ridges, we employed IMT, a quantitative method to assess individual sweat gland activity to secrete sweat. All participants were tested for sweating responses in an air-conditioned room maintained between 22.0 and 24.0°C at 40–50% relative humidity (RH), and were allowed to acclimate to this temperature and RH for at least 30 min prior to the study (baseline measurement). Sweating was induced by immersing both legs for 15–30 min in a water bath maintained at 43°C, as described previously [7]. In addition to this, we also employed two different experimental trials to induce sweating: exposure to high ambient humidity (80% RH) or increased temperature (28°C). The two experimental trials were chosen to elicit sufficiently large sweating responses based on the results of preliminary experiments. During these trials, skin temperature was measured at sites in which sweating responses were measured. In addition to employing IMT, the degree of sweating responses was partly determined by measuring the SSH at different time points before and after starting thermal stimulus [7].

As shown in figure 2a, in IMT sweat droplets were largely detected at the folds even under quiescent conditions before thermal stimulus, although much less in number as compared with those after thermal stimulus. This finding indicates that basal levels of sweating ('insensible' sweating) occur in an unrecognized fashion and suggests that the SSH levels under quiescent basal conditions may reflect such basal levels of sweating from glands/ducts located at the folds. To in-

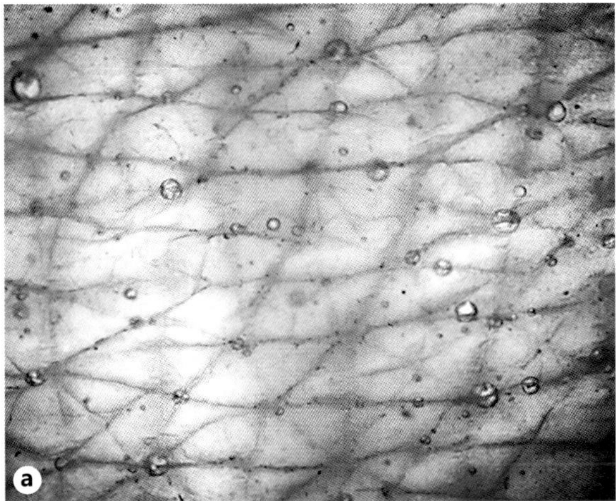

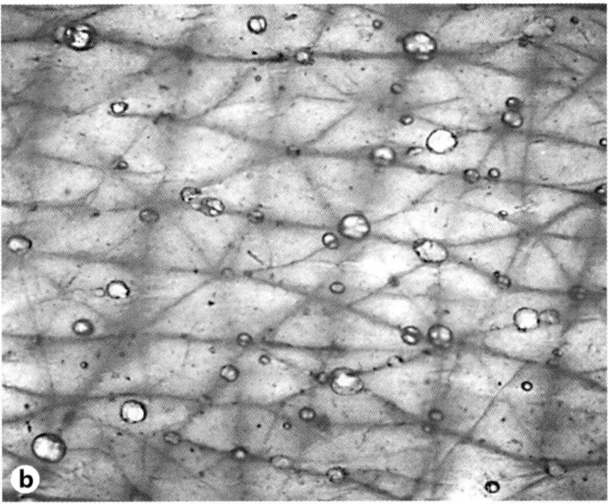

Fig. 2. Sweating responses in healthy subjects evaluated by IMT before (**a**) and 30 min after (**b**) thermal stimulus.

vestigate this possibility, we asked whether there could be an association between the SSH status and the number or size of sweat droplets detected either at the folds or ridges under quiescent conditions. A positive correlation was only found between the SSH status and number of sweat droplets detected at the folds, but not those at the ridges. A likely interpretation of these findings is that sweating responses in sweat ducts/glands located at the folds in hairy skin function as natural regulators that can maintain skin hydration under basal conditions (fig. 3).

We next investigated whether thermal stimulus could increase the number of sweat droplets located either at the folds or ridges. As shown in figure 2b, a marked increase in the number of sweat droplets was preferentially observed in sweat glands/ducts located at the ridges 30 min after thermal stimulus, although a smaller increase in the number of sweat droplets was also observed in sweat glands/ducts located at the folds. Importantly, there was no significant rise in skin temperature after thermal stimulus as compared with the basal measurement: skin temperature remained fairly constant during thermal stimulus by immersion of legs in warm water.

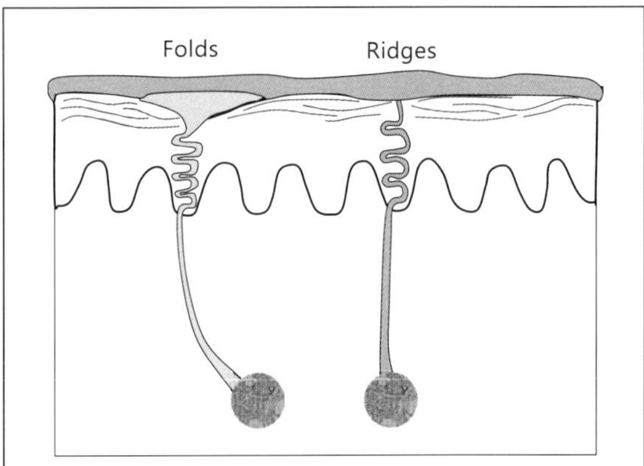

Fig. 3. Difference in the function of sweat glands depending on their anatomical location. Sweat glands located at the folds serve to maintain SSH. In contrast, those located at the folds serve as a thermoregulator or backup to those at the folds.

These results suggest that sweat glands/ducts located at the ridges might function as key thermoregulators unlike those at the folds.

Indeed, such a marked increase in the number of sweat droplets located at the ridges was never observed after exposure either to high humidity (80% RH) or warm ambient temperature (28°C), although there was a minimal increase in the number of sweat droplets located at the folds [Sato et al., manuscript submitted]. Importantly, this minimal increase in the number of sweat droplets located at the folds was associated with the rise in skin temperature. These results clearly indicate that the immersion of legs in warm water is much more efficient for both inducing sweat from sweat glands/ducts located at the ridges and increasing the sweating rate without causing temperature rise. Thus, the maintenance of 'insensible' sweating from glands/ducts located at the folds is critical for maintaining stratum corneum moisture content. In contrast, sweating responses of sweat ducts located at the ridges seem to have a more dramatic effect on thermoregulation than those at the folds. In the next section, we focus on a group of inflammatory skin diseases that may be caused by sweating disturbances.

Sweat Gland-/Duct-Related Skin Disease

Atopic Dermatitis

Although Sato et al. [13] summarized the disorders of eccrine sweating, this list is just the tip of the iceberg. As Sato et al. [10, 13] described, our knowledge of normal and abnormal eccrine sweat gland physiology is still in its infancy. The spectrum of sweat gland-/duct-related skin diseases would be expanded by the identification of diseases which are caused by extravasated sweat in the dermis or epidermis. In this regard, sweating disturbances may provide exciting new clues to our understanding of AD because there have been conflicting data regarding whether sweating responses are impaired, normal, or enhanced in patients with AD. These conflicting results suggest that there is more to be learned about the disturbance of sweating.

We therefore investigated how disease processes and sweating disturbance progress from early asymptomatic stages through to the onset of clinically apparent disease. To elucidate how the disease progresses in association with sweating defects, AD patients were divided into two types based on the clinical phenotypes and stages: acute and chronic. Patients with active dermatitis characterized by scaling erythematous papules, plaques, lichenoid papules, and crusting were defined as acute AD: most of them had exudate lesions in the flexural areas, usually for <5 years. In contrast, patients characterized by systemic dry skin and relative sparing of eczematous lesions in the flexural area were defined as chronic AD. Importantly, the number of sweat droplets detected at the folds was profoundly decreased even in normal-appearing uninvolved skin at early asymptomatic stages, where skin surface structures had not been disrupted, indicating that sweating defects may develop before clinically apparent skin lesions appear. In this normal-appearing uninvolved skin, there was a high degree of variability in the number and size of sweat droplets, ranging from a simple reduction in number to the appearance of large sizes of sweat droplets, the latter of which would represent the earliest, but asymptomatic, AD lesions (data not shown).

The number of sweat droplets located at the folds in the involved skin of acute AD, but not those at the ridges (fig. 4a), was apparently lower than that in healthy controls. Interestingly, the decrease in the number of sweat droplets located at the folds was associated with the increase in the size of sweat droplets located at the ridges (fig. 4a). This result suggests that compensatory hyperhidrosis preferentially occurs in sweat glands/ducts at the ridges. As the disease process evolves, this compensatory hyperhidrosis became blurred. In the chronic stage of AD, systemic hypohidrosis characterized by a profound decrease in the number of sweat droplets was observed either at the folds or the ridges (fig. 4b), and could contribute to the progression of the disease process to the full development of AD characterized by systemic dry skin.

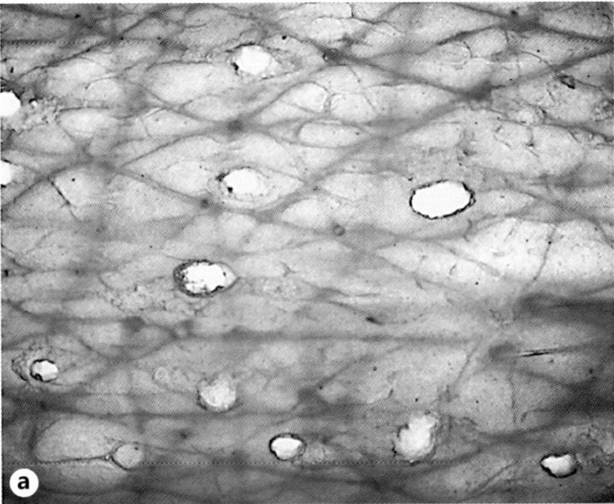

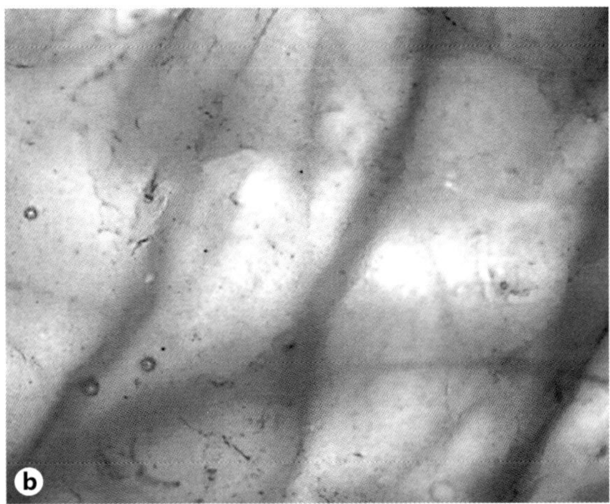

Fig. 4. Sweating responses in acute and chronic AD evaluated by IMT 30 min after thermal stimulus. A profound decrease in the number of sweat droplets at the folds can be observed. **a** The decrease is associated with the increase in the size of sweat droplets located at the ridges, indicating compensatory hyperhidrosis. **b** In chronic AD, the number and size of sweat droplets located either at the folds or the ridges are markedly decreased.

One important question would be whether a decrease in sweating responses could be due to their inability to produce sweat or to deliver sweat to the skin surface. Because DCD peptides are sweat-specific components but not the components common to other body fluids [3], we investigated whether DCD peptides could be immunohistochemically detected in the sweat glands/ducts of AD patients as detected in those in healthy controls. In the biopsy specimens taken from the involved skin of acute AD before thermal stimulus, DCD was abundantly detected in the cytoplasm of dark cells in the sweat glands at a higher intensity than that in those of healthy controls and those of psoriasis vulgaris (PV) lesions, indicating that the decreased sweating observed in AD patients is not due to their inability to produce sweat, but may be due to their inability to deliver sweat to the surface. However, there were no keratotic plugs that can obstruct normal sweat delivery in any AD lesions.

We next asked the alternative possibility that sweat may seep from the damaged epithelial lining of the sweat ducts in the absence of real blockage, due to sweat duct fragility, as observed in the stratum corneum of AD patients. To this end, biopsy specimens were also obtained from the involved skin after thermal stimulus. Surprisingly, DCD was detected not only in the sweat glands/ducts, but also in the dermal tissue adjacent to the glands and ducts [Shimoda et al., manuscript submitted]. Such leakage of sweat into the dermis near the ducts was never detected in PV lesions even after thermal stimulus. These results indicate that sweat could diffuse into the dermal tissue around the glands/ducts due to sweat duct fragility, and the delivery of sweat into the surface could be impaired as a consequence of the sweat leakage. Such diffusion of sweat into the dermis would represent the early event that triggers the recruitment and activation of immune cells. In view of the fact that sweat has been shown to have various inflammatory cytokines [14–16], it is likely that leakage of sweat into the dermis could initiate a complex sequence of events that promotes eczematous inflammation. Given the previous finding that the areas of anhidrosis on thermoregulatory sweat testing correspond to their symptomatic areas, such as itching and strange sensation [17], the itching and strange sensation that AD patients frequently complain about when sweating can now alternatively be explained by such leakage of sweat into the dermis rather than by small-fiber neuropathy proposed by the authors.

Numerous animal models of AD have been described, including chemically induced AD-like chromic dermatitis [17, 18], inbred animal strains [19, 20], and knockout animals [21, 22]. These models are useful for investigating the pathophysiology of skin inflammation. However, since these studies have been performed in skin devoid of sweat glands/ducts, one should be cautious in interpreting these findings as the actual disease model. Indeed, animals with targeted manipulations of the recently identified AD susceptibility genes do not necessarily develop a clear AD phenotype [21]. Such findings may be partly explained by the lack of sweat glands/ducts in the hairy skin of these animals, in which investigations have been performed.

Here we propose that the pathogenesis of AD occurs in three temporally overlapping stages. First is the initial stage, in which leakage of sweat into the dermis in some areas due to sweat duct fragility not only serves to initiate the inflammatory response, but also results in the profound decrease in SSH. Second is the compensatory stage, in which compensatory hyperhidrosis occurs preferentially at the ridges to maintain thermoregulation, which further exacerbates the inflammatory response. Third is a 'burn-out' process in later stages, in which patients eventually manifest the phenotype with a systemic disturbance in the sweat delivery system not associated with compensatory hyperhidrosis. This model suggests that one might be able to interrupt this process by therapies directed at correcting sweating defects at early stages.

Little is known about the possibility that therapeutic agents presently available to treat AD, such as topical corticosteroids, may drive sweating defects forward. Although no major adverse effects of topical corticosteroids on the function of sweat glands/ducts have been reported, we are concerned that protracted use of topical corticosteroids may exert potentially detrimental effects on sweat glands/ducts which could persist long after the drug is withdrawn. Although sweating defects observed in AD is unlikely to be exclusively induced by the direct effect of topical corticosteroids on sweat glands/ducts, our ongoing experiments with the use of IMT show that treatment with topical corticosteroids for 1 week in normal skin of healthy controls reduced the number of sweat droplets while a topical moisturizer for 1 week markedly increased the number of sweat droplets, especially those at the folds. In contrast, traditional emollients, such as Vaseline, reduced the number of sweat droplets when used for 1 week. These results suggest that a favorable clinical benefit could be anticipated with treatment with a moisturizer, but not an emollient, for sweat gland-/duct-related disease refractory to corticosteroids, probably by which sweat delivery to the skin surface could be made easier.

Lichen Planus and Other Lichenoid Diseases

Because the early phase of lesion development in lichen planus (LP) and other lichenoid diseases is characterized by T-cell infiltration in the upper dermis, the majority of the clinical and experimental work on LP has focused on T cells while ignoring the identification and characterization of an upstream signal that facilitates the highly directed migration of the pathogenic T cells to inflammatory lesions. Thus, it remains unknown how the pathogenic T cells are recruited to specific tissues.

In this regard, earlier studies by Akosa and Lampert [23, 24] could give an important clue as to the identification of the upstream signal: they demonstrated sweat gland abnormalities in LP and other lichenoid dermatoses more than 20 years ago; however, their studies have received little attention. These studies prompted us to in-

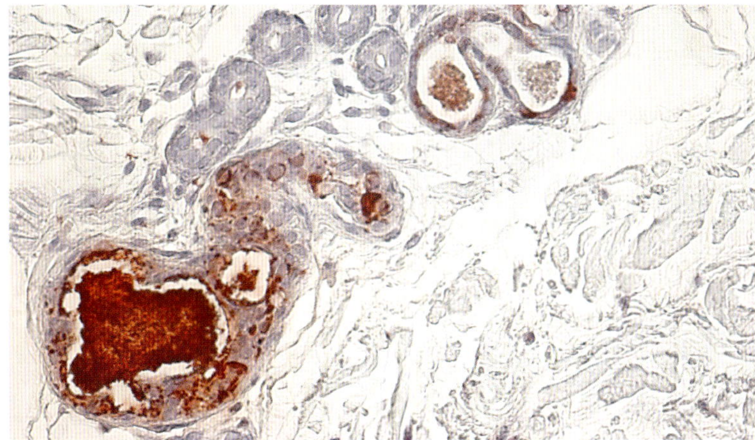

Fig. 5. Immunohistochemical detection of DCD indicating retention of sweat in the eccrine glands of LP lesions.

vestigate whether sweat gland abnormalities could represent an early event in the development of skin inflammation in these diseases or a secondary event. Our recent studies have also demonstrated that sweat retention can be specifically observed in the eccrine sweat glands of active lesions of LP (fig. 5), but not in PV, and suggested that sweating disturbances could be responsible for the development of LP lesions [25]. Consistent with this view, an earlier study by Sato et al. [10, 13] predicted that eccrine sweat can modify various dematoses if sweat diffuses into the epidermis.

We therefore quantitatively evaluated sweating responses to thermal stimulus in the involved and perilesional uninvolved areas of LP and PV patients and healthy controls by determining the number of active sweat glands/ducts and the volume of the sweat. In the involved area of LP, a marked decrease in the number of sweat droplets was observed: the complete absence of sweat droplets was observed in either the earliest phase of LP lesions or established lesions, while compensatory increases in the number or size of sweat droplets were never detected in the neighboring uninvolved area, unlike a finding in AD in which compensatory hyperhidrosis could be detected in the peripheral uninvolved area. Even in the perilesional skin of LP, a significant decrease in the number of sweat droplets was specifically observed, but not in the peripheral skin lesions of PV: a pinpoint loss of sweat droplets was abundantly detected in the normal-appearing perilesional skin of LP. The profound decrease in the size was also noted in LP lesions. Thus, sweat volume per square centimeter calculated from the number and size of sweat droplets was profoundly decreased in the LP lesions, regardless of the age of the lesions. More importantly, a marked, pinpoint loss of sweat droplets, which we refer to as a 'cold spot', was also observed in the uninvolved perilesional skin. Surprisingly, the cold spot area was clinically invisible at the time of IMT, but became lesional within 2–3 days without any treatment. In contrast, the appearance of cold spots was minimal in the uninvolved peripheral skin of PV, although a profound decrease in sweat droplets was also observed in the involved skin of PV.

To further confirm that the appearance of such cold spots represents the actual early event needed for the subsequent development of the clinical LP lesions, we attempted to determine whether leakage of sweat that can cause inflammation could be specifically observed in the cold spot areas. DCD was expressed in the cytoplasm

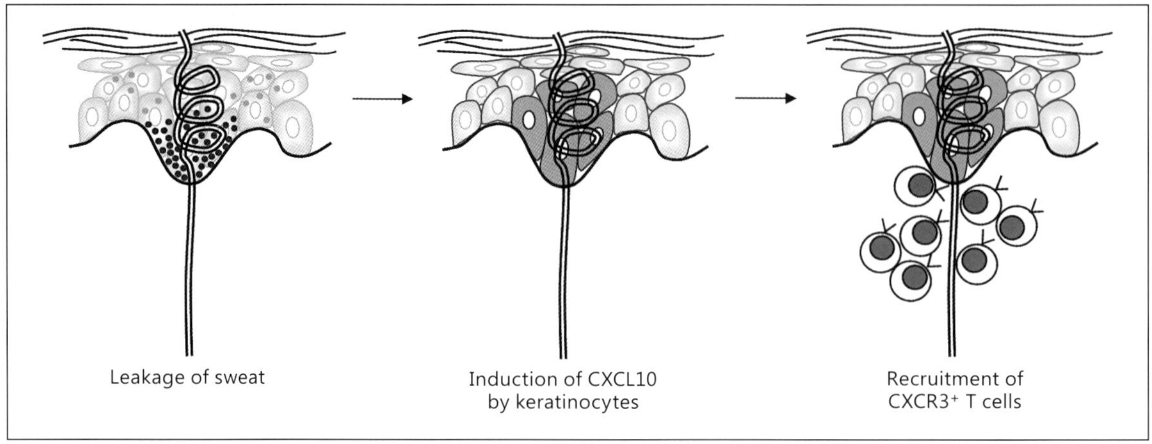

Fig. 6. Hypothetical model for LP. Selective migration of CXCR3$^+$ T cells to the epidermis expressing CXCL10 can be initially triggered by leakage of sweat into the acrosyringium.

of dark cells and luminal membranes of eccrine glands, but not in the ducts. When compared with the staining intensity in other inflammatory diseases, such as PV, DCD immunoreactivity of sweat glands was greatest in LP lesions (fig. 5) and least in PV lesions. Strong staining for DCD was also detected in amorphous intraluminal materials seen in the enlarged lumen of the glands and ducts, suggesting retention of sweat.

These findings suggest that the sweat glands in LP lesions have sufficient ability to produce sweat, but the ability to deliver sweat to the skin surface could be impaired, probably due to blockage of the duct or duct fragility as observed in AD. To test this possibility, serial sections obtained from the cold spots in normal-appearing perilesional skin of LP after thermal stimulus were immunohistochemically stained for DCD expression. DCD expression was not only detected in the sweat glands, but also in the intraluminal materials up to the portion around the epidermal/dermal junction. Surprisingly, it was also specifically detected within the epidermis restricted to the portion (acrosyringium) around the eccrine ducts. DCD expression in such an acrosyringium-restricted manner was never detected in AD and PV lesions, even after thermal stimulus.

Of importance, the expression of DCD around the acrosyringium was associated with expression of CXCL10 by surrounding keratinocytes and accumulation of CXCR3$^+$ T cells beneath the epidermis [Mizukawa, manuscript submitted]. Those results indicate that leakage of sweat around the acrosyringium represent the actual early event that can trigger selective migration of CXCR3$^+$ T cells directed towards the intraepidermal portion of the eccrine ducts through the induction of CXCL10 in keratinocytes (fig. 6). Among a variety of chemokines, CXCL10 has recently been suggested to play an important role for attracting pathogenic T cells in various autoimmune diseases such as rheumatoid arthritis [26]. In addition to the role for T-cell chemotaxis, serum CXCL10 levels have been suggested to be useful biomarkers predictive of progression to severe epidermal damage [27] and for the management of patients with several inflammatory diseases including chronic hepatitis [28]. A consensus has emerged from recent studies [29, 30] that CXCR3 and CCR5 preferentially expressed on effector memory T cells are cell-surface chemokine receptors that guide the T cells to inflammatory sites while CXCR4 and CCR7 are associated with constitutive migration of T cells through lymph nodes. Thus, the functional relevance of the CXCR3-CXCL10 pathway has been extensively confirmed in various inflammatory diseases and experimental models. Because recent studies have demonstrated that normal human sweat contains proteolytic enzymes, IL-1α, IL-1β, IL-6, IL-8, IL-31, TNF-α, and epidermal growth factor [31–34], some of which have been shown to induce leukocyte recruitment to the skin, the proinflammatory recruitment of T cells would be further amplified by the leakage of sweat in the epidermal-dermal junction.

It remains unknown why leakage of sweat occurs at different portions of sweat ducts in AD and LP: in AD sweat leaks at the dermal duct while in LP sweat migrates into the intraepidermal duct (acrosyringium). Then, the question arises whether sweat ducts could have different barrier systems depending on the portion. Indeed, a difference in the expression of the tight junction (TJ)-associated proteins such as occludin, claudin 1, and claudin 4 between the dermal ducts and intraepidermal ducts has been reported: the dermal ducts show a colocalization of occludin and claudin 4, but lack a protective layer of cornified corneocytes, while the intraepidermal ducts show no colocalization of occludin and claudin 1 or claudin 4, and lack a functional TJ [35]. As a consequence, the barrier built in the intraepidermal ducts would be not as tight as the dermal ducts built in the TJ. Thus, the acrosyringium could have an alternative barrier system other than the TJ, which would be functionally impaired in LP and lichenoid diseases. In view of previous reports describing the development of LP after resolution of herpes zoster [36], viral infection may alter the function of the barrier system built in the acrosyringium. In support of this possibility, our unpublished observations indicate that the occurrence of localized hypohidrosis is a common event during and after onset of herpes zoster [Ushigome et al., manuscript submitted], although many of these patients have not recognized the localized hypohidrosis.

Thus, because extravasated sweat can cause epidermal damage due to the diffusion of proteolytic enzymes in sweat, lichenoid lymphocytic infiltrates observed in many lichenoid skin diseases could be triggered by such leakage of sweat into the dermal-epidermal junction or dermis. Indeed, a sweating disturbance as observed in LP was also detected in the papules of lichen amyloidosis (LA) and purpura pigmentosa chronica [Shimoda et al., manuscript submitted].

Management of Sweat Gland-/Duct-Related Diseases

Treatment of these sweat gland-/duct-related diseases, such as LP and LA, is extremely difficult and no modalities have produced complete resolution without a subsequent relapse of disease. In most patients, a combination of different treatment modalities including topical corticosteroids, oral cyclosporine, and phototherapy is needed to achieve a long-lasting effect. These eruptions are largely refractory to long-term treatment with topical corticosteroids and phototherapy.

We asked whether a moisturizer, heparinoid, could improve these eruptions refractory to various treatment modalities including topical corticosteroids because our unpublished study clearly demonstrated that a topical moisturizer for 1 week, when used in an aggressively high dose or under occlusion, markedly increased the number of sweat droplets, especially those at the folds. In LA, LP, and purpura pigmentosa chronica, a remarkable increase in the number of sweat droplets was detected 1–2 weeks after starting therapy with a moisturizer and the increase was associated with the restoration of skin surface patterns under basal conditions before thermal stimulus. In particular, treatment with a moisturizer under occlusive dressing produced complete resolution of these eruptions associated with increased sweating reposes after thermal stimulus. Histological analyses of the resolved LA lesions disclosed elimination of amyloid deposition, which was associated with the appearance of pore opening in the 'hub' corresponding to the center of LA papules. The leakage or retention of sweat frequently observed in nontreated LA lesions was never detected in the completely resolved LA lesions treated with a moisturizer under occlusive dressing. Thus, our results clearly show that treatment of sweat gland-/duct-related disease should be primarily directed at preventing the leakage of sweat into the epidermis or dermis by which sweat delivery to the skin surface could be made easier. The sweating disturbances observed in these diseases could be restored by a moisturizer, particularly under occlusion.

Conclusion

A list of sweat gland-/duct-related diseases would expand more and more if dermatologists could recognize sweating disturbance as an etiologic factor involved in the development of these skin diseases refractory to conventional therapies. The disease process would begin weeks or months before the development of clinically apparent diseases. Because leakage of sweat into the epidermis or dermis, although necessary for the induction of lesions, does not necessarily become a lesion, there is probably a second event in the skin which is needed for complete evolution of the clinically apparent skin lesions. Much work remains to further evaluate our concept presented here.

Acknowledgement

This work was supported in part by grants from the Ministry of Education, Culture, Sports, Science and Technology (to T.S.) and the Health and Labour Sciences Research Grants (Research on Intractable Diseases) from the Ministry of Health, Labour and Welfare of Japan (to T.S.).

References

1 Morren MA, Przybilla B, Bamelis M, Heykants B, Reynaers A, Degreef H: Atopic dermatitis: triggering factors. J Am Acad Dermatol 1994;31:467–473.
2 Kusunoki T, Asai K, Harazaki M, Korematsu S, Hosoi S: Month of birth and prevalence of atopic dermatitis in schoolchildren: dry skin in early infancy as a possible etiologic factor. J Allergy Clin Immunol 1999;103:1148–1152.
3 Rieg S, Seeber S, Steffen H, Humeny A, Kalbacher H, Stevanovic S, Kimura A, Garbe C, Schittek B: Generation of multiple stable dermcidin-derived antimicrobial peptides in sweat of different body sites. J Invest Dermatol 2006;126: 354–365.
4 Watanabe A, Sugawara T, Kikuchi K, Yamasaki K, Sakai S, Aiba S: Sweat constitutes several natural moisturizing factors, lactate, urea, sodium, and potassium. J Dermatol Sci 2013;72:177–182.
5 Boguniewicz M, Leung DY: Atopic dermatitis: a disease of altered skin barrier and immune dysregulation. Immunol Rev 2011;242:233–246.
6 Palmer CN, Irvine AD, Terron-Kwiatkowski A, Zhao Y, Liao H, Lee SP, et al: Common loss-of-function variants of the epidermal barrier protein filaggrin are a major predisposing factor for atopic dermatitis. Nat Genet 2006;38:441–446.
7 Shiohara T, Doi T, Hayakawa J: Defective sweating responses in atopic dermatitis. Curr Probl Dermatol 2011;41:68–79.
8 Nattkemper LA, Lee HG, Vades-Rodriguez R, Mollanazar NK, Sanders KM, Yosipovitch G: Cholinergic induction of perspiration attenuates nonhistaminergic pruritus in the skin of patients with atopic dermatitis and healthy controls. Br J Dermatol 2015;173:282–284.
9 Groscurth P: Anatomy of sweat glands. Curr Probl Dermatol 2002;30:1–9.
10 Sato K, Kang WH, Saga K, Sato KT: Biology of sweat glands and their disorders. I. Normal sweat gland function. J Am Acad Dermatol 1989;20:537–563.
11 Asahina M, Poudel A, Hirano S: Sweating on the palm and sole: physiological and clinical relevance. Clin Auton Res 2015;25:153–159.
12 Cui CY, Schlessinger D: Eccrine sweat gland development and sweat secretion. Exp Dermatol 2015;24:644–650.

13 Sato K, Kang WH, Saga K, Sato KT: Biology of sweat glands and their disorders. II. Disorders of sweat gland function. J Am Acad Dermatol 1989;20:713–726.
14 Ahmed AA, Nordlind K, Schultzberg M, Lidén S: Proinflammatory cytokines and their corresponding receptor proteins in eccrine sweat glands in normal and cutaneous leishmaniasis human skin. An immunohistochemical study. Exp Dermatol 1996;5:230–235.
15 Marques-Deak A, Cizza G, Eskandari F, Torvik S, Christie IC, et al: Measurement of cytokines in sweat patches and plasma in healthy women: validation in a controlled study. J Immunol Methods 2006;315:99–109.
16 Dai X, Okazaki H, Hanakawa Y, Murakami M, Tohyama M, Shirakata Y, Sayama K: Eccrine sweat contains IL-1α, IL1β and IL-31 and activates epidermal keratinocytes as a danger signal. PLoS One 2013;8:e67666.
17 Kitagaki H, Kimishima M, Teraki Y, Hayakawa J, Hayakawa K, Fujisawa S, Shiohara T: Distinct in vivo and in vitro cytokine profiles of draining lymph node cells in acute and chronic phases of contact hypersensitivity: importance of a type 2 cytokine-rich cutaneous milieu for the development of an early-type response in the chronic phase. J Immunol 1999;163:1265–1273.
18 Kitagaki H, Hiyama H, Kitazawa T, Shiohara T: Psychological stress with long-standing allergic dermatitis causes psychodermatological conditions in mice. J Invest Dermatol 2014;134:1561–1569.
19 Matsumoto M, Ra C, Kawamoto K, Sato H, Itakura A, Sawada J, Ushio H, Suto H, Mitsuishi K, Hikasa Y, Matsuda H: IgE hyperproduction through enhanced tyrosine phosphorylation of Janus kinase 3 in NC/Nga mice, a model for human atopic dermatitis. J Immunol 1999;162:1056–1063.
20 Vercelli D: Of flaky tails and itchy skin. Nat Genet 2009;41:512–513.
21 Sasaki T, Shiohama A, Kubo A, Kawasaki H, Ishida-Yamamoto A, Yamada T, Hachiya T, Shimizu A, Okano H, Kudoh J, Amagai M: A homozygous nonsense mutation in the gene for Tmem79, a component for experimental models of atopic dermatitis. J Allergy Clin Immunol 2013;132,1111–1120.
22 Saunders SP, Goh CS, Brown SJ, Palmer CN, Porter RM, Cole C, Fallon PG, et al: Tmem79/Matt is the matted mouse gene and is a predisposing gene for atopic dermatitis in human subjects. J Allergy Clin Immunol 2013;132:1121–1129.
23 Akosa AB, Lampert IA: The sweat gland in graft versus host disease. J Pathol 1990;161:261–266.
24 Akosa AB, Lampert IA: Sweat gland abnormalities in lichenoid dermatosis. Histopathology 1991;19:345–349.
25 Horie C, Mizukawa Y, Shiohara T: Histological evaluation of sweat glands and ducts in lichenoid tissue reaction (in Japanese). Jpn J Dermatol 2011;121:1869–1874.
26 Antonelli A, Ferrari SM, Giuggioli D, Ferrannini E, Ferri C, Fallahi P: Chemokine (C-X-C motif) ligand (CXCL) 10 in autoimmune diseases. Autoimmun Rev 2014;13:272–280.
27 Shiohara T, Mizukawa Y, Aoyama Y: Monitoring the acute response in severe hypersensitivity reactions to drugs. Curr Opin Allergy Clin Immunol 2015;15:294–299.
28 Casrouge A, Bisiaux A, Stephen L, Schmolz M, Mapes J, Pfister C, Pol S, Mallet V, Albert ML: Discrimination of agonist and antagonist forms of CXCL10 in biological samples. Clin Exp Immunol 2012;167:137–148.
29 Iijima W, Ohtani H, Nakayama T, Sugawara Y, Sato E, Nagura H, Yoshie O, Sasano T: Infiltrating CD8+ T cells in oral lichen planus predominantly express CCR5 and CXCR3 and carry respective chemokine ligands RANTES/CCL5 and IP-10/CXCL10 in their cytolytic granules: a potential self-recruiting mechanism. Am J Pathol 2003;163:261–268.
30 Wenzel J, Tüting T: An IFN-associated cytotoxic cellular immune response against viral, self-, or tumor antigens is a common pathogenetic feature in 'interface dermatitis'. J Invest Dermatol 2008;128:2392–2402.
31 Sato K, Sato F: Interleukin-1 alpha in human sweat is functionally active and derived from the eccrine sweat gland. Am J Physiol 1994;266:R950–R959.
32 Jones AP, Webb LM, Anderson AO, Leonard EJ, Rot A: Normal human sweat contains interleukin-8. J Leukoc Biol 1995;57:434–437.
33 Li HH, Zhou G, Fu XB, Zhang L: Antigen expression of human eccrine sweat glands. J Cutan Pathol 2009;36:318–324.
34 Dai X, Okazaki H, Hanakawa Y, Murakami M, Tohyama M, Shirakata Y, Sayama K: Eccrine sweat contains IL-1α, IL-1β and IL-31 and activates epidermal keratinocytes as a danger signal. PLoS One 2013;8:e67666.
35 Wilke K, Wepf R, Keil FJ, Wittern KP, Wenck H, Biel SS: Are sweat glands an alternate penetration pathway? Understanding the morphological complexity of the axillary sweat gland apparatus. Skin Pharmacol Physiol 2006;19:38–49.
36 Mizukawa Y, Horie C, Yamazaki Y, Shiohara T: Detection of varicella-zoster virus antigens in lesional skin of zosteriform lichen planus but not in that of linear lichen planus. Dermatology 2012;225:22–26.

Tetsuo Shiohara, MD, PhD
Department of Dermatology
Kyorin University School of Medicine
6-20-2 Shinkawa, Mitaka
Tokyo 181-8611 (Japan)
E-Mail tpshio@ks.kyorin-u.ac.jp

Yokozeki H, Murota H, Katayama I (eds): Perspiration Research.
Curr Probl Dermatol. Basel, Karger, 2016, vol 51, pp 42–49 (DOI: 10.1159/000446757)

Genetic Disorders with Dyshidrosis: Ectodermal Dysplasia, Incontinentia Pigmenti, Fabry Disease, and Congenital Insensitivity to Pain with Anhidrosis

Mari Wataya-Kaneda

Department of Dermatology, Graduate School of Medicine, Osaka University, Osaka, Japan

Abstract

Sweating is regulated by various neurohormonal mechanisms. A disorder in any part of the sweating regulatory pathways, such as the thermal center, neurotransmitters in the central to peripheral nerve, innervation of periglandular neurotransmission, and sweat secretion in the sweat gland itself, induces dyshidrosis. Therefore, hereditary disorders with dyshidrosis result from a variety of causes. These diseases have characteristic symptoms derived from each pathogenesis besides dyshidrosis. The information in this chapter is useful for the differential diagnosis of representative genetic disorders with dyshidrosis.

Various neurohormonal mechanisms regulate sweating. When cutaneous C fibers in a localized area of the skin are activated by an increase in temperature, the preoptic hypothalamus area is activated and provides the stimulation for sweat production. The activated hypothalamus area provokes the sympathetic postganglionic fibers surrounding the sweat glands and stimulates the eccrine sweat glands with acetylcholine, which is the principal terminal neurotransmitter contrary to the ordinary sympathetic innervation, to induce sweating.

A disorder in any part of the sweating regulatory pathways, such as the thermal center, neurotransmitters in the central to peripheral nerve, innervation of periglandular neurotransmission and sweat secretion in the sweat gland itself, induces dyshidrosis, and there are many hereditary diseases involving dyshidrosis. In this chapter, representative genetic disorders with dyshidrosis, including ectodermal dysplasia (ED), incontinentia pigmenti (IP), Fabry disease, and congenital insensitivity to pain with anhidrosis (CIPA) are discussed.

Ectodermal Dysplasia

One of the representative diseases is ED, which is a hereditary heterogeneous syndrome characterized by anomalies in the structures and functions of ectodermal origin. Thurnam [1] first described

Table 1. Genotype and phenotype (include sweating) of ED

	Gene	Pathway	Disease	Inheritance
ED-EDAR-EDARADD signaling pathway	*ED-1*	Ectodysplasin/ectodysplasin-A	Anhidrotic ED	XL
	EDAR	Ectodysplasin/ectodysplasin-A receptor	Anhidrotic ED	AD, AR
	EDARADD	EDAR-associated death domain	Anhidrotic ED	AR
NEMO regulatory pathway	*NEMO/IκKγ*	NF-κB	Anhidrotic ED with immunodeficiency	XL
			Anhidrotic ED with osteopetrosis and immunodeficiency	XL
			IP	XL
	IκBα	IKNα	Anhidrotic ED with immunodeficiency	AD
Abnormal interaction between the ectoderm and the mesenchyme	*p63*	p63	EEC syndrome	AD
			AEC syndrome	AD
			ADULT syndrome	AD
			Limb-mammary syndrome	AD
			Rapp-Hodgkin syndrome	AD
	DLX3	DLX3	Tricho-dento-osseous syndrome	AD
	MSX1	MSX1	Witkop disease	AD
	EVC2	EVC2	Ellis-van Creveld disease	AD
	EVC	EVC	Weyers acrodental dysostosis	AD
			Ellis-van Creveld disease	AR
Abnormalities in tissue homeostasis and growth control	*WNT10A*	WNT10A	Odonto-onycho-dermal dysplasia	AR
	GJB6	Connexin30	Clouston syndrome	AD
	PVRL1	Nectin1	ED with cleft lip/palate	AD
	PKP1	Plakophilin 1	ED with fragile skin syndrome	AR
	CDH3	Cadherin 3	ED with ectrodactyly and macular dystrophy	AR

AD = Autosomal dominant transmission; ADULT = acro-dermato-ungual-lacrimal-tooth; AEC = ankyloblepharon-ED-cleft lip/palate; AR = autosomal recessive transmission; EEC = ectrodactyly, ED, and cleft lip/palate; XL = X-linked.

ED in 1948. The estimated incidence is 7 in 10,000 births. To date, approximately 30 causative genes have been identified. The classification of ED is complex, and explanations of clinical and genetic data regarding ED have been attempted [2, 3].

Two groups of ED have been distinguished [4]. One is characterized by aplasia or hypoplasia of the ectodermal tissues, which fails to develop and differentiate because of a lack of reciprocal signaling between the ectoderm and mesoderm. This group is further subdivided into 2 groups [5]. One group involves the signaling pathway that modulates the activity of nuclear factor kappa B (NF-κB), which includes the EDA (ectodysplasin/ectodysplasin-A)-EDAR (ectodysplasin/ectodysplasin-A receptor)-EDARADD (ectodysplasin/ectodysplasin-A receptor-associated death domain)-NEMO (NF-κB essential modulator) regulatory pathway, and is related to regulatory changes in the transcription and/or expression of genes such as p63/TP63 (tumor protein p63), *DLX3* (distal-less homeobox 3), *MSX1* (msh homeobox 1), *EVC2* (Ellis-van Creveld syndrome 2), and *EVC* (Ellis-van Creveld syndrome).

The other group corresponds to the abnormal function of structural proteins in the cell membrane, such as nectin 1, connexins, plakophilin, cadherin, and Wnt10A. These are characterized by a skin abnormality, such as palmoplantar keratoderma, as their most striking feature, with or without deafness or retinal dystrophy.

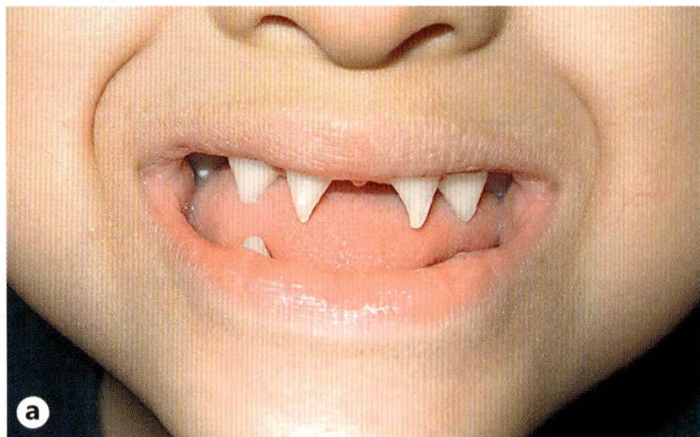

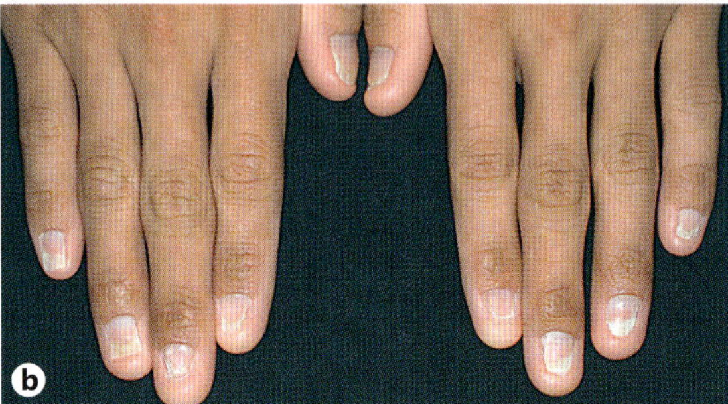

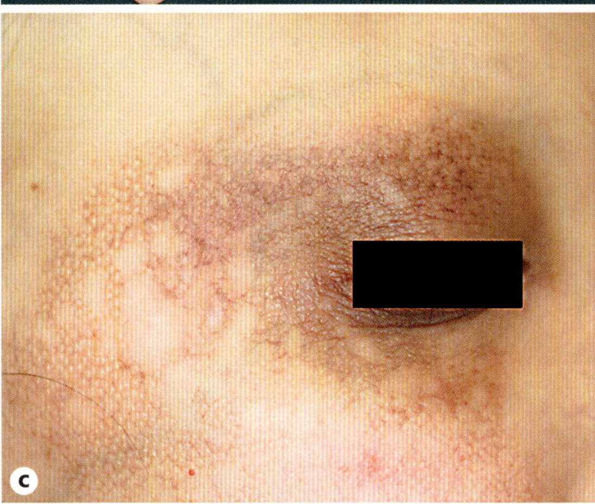

Fig. 1. Clinical manifestations of ED. A reduced number of teeth (hypodontia) and malformation of the teeth (**a**), nail dysplasia (**b**), and darkly pigmented and wrinkled skin around the eyes (**c**) are present.

ED is also divided into 2 major types of disorders based on clinical findings, such as sweating, hypohidrotic or anhidrotic ED (H/AED) in which sweat glands are either absent or significantly reduced in number, and hidrotic ED in which sweat glands are normal and the condition is inherited in an autosomal dominant manner. Although many genes are involved in ED as described above, only 4 genes, *EDA1*, *EDAR*, *EDARADD*, and *WNT10A*, account for 90% of H/AED cases [6]. The related genes, genotypes, and phenotypes (sweating) of ED are summarized in table 1.

H/AED is characterized by the abnormal development of organs of ectodermal origin, such as sweat glands, teeth, nails, and hair, and is estimated to occur in approximately 1 in 5,000–10,000 newborns. H/AED is primarily characterized by the partial or complete absence of certain sweat glands (eccrine glands), causing a lack of or diminished sweating, heat intolerance, and fever, and the absence of or abnormally sparse hair (hypotrichosis), or the absence of or a decreased number of teeth (adontia/hypodontia) and/or the malformation of teeth (fig. 1a). Many individuals with H/AED also have characteristic facial abnormalities, including a prominent forehead, a sunken nasal bridge ('saddle nose'), unusually thick lips, and/or a large chin. The skin on most of the body may be abnormally thin, dry, soft, and hypopigmented. However, the skin around the eyes may be darkly pigmented and finely wrinkled (fig. 1c). In many cases, the affected infants and children may also exhibit hypoplasia or aplasia of the mucous glands within the respiratory and gastrointestinal tracts, and in some cases decreased functions of the immune system, such as depressed lymphocyte function and, rarely, decreased cellular immunity. This potentially causes an increased susceptibility to certain infections and/or allergic conditions. Many affected infants and children experience recurrent attacks of wheezing and asthma, respiratory infections, chronic inflammation of the nasal passages (atrophic rhinitis), scaling, itchy skin rashes (eczema), and/or other findings.

X-linked HED is the most frequent form of H/AED, with an incidence of approximately 1 per 100,000 births [7]. It occurs as a result of mutations in the *ED1* gene, also known as *EDA* [8].

Although patients with X-linked H/AED display typical symptoms, the characteristic findings do not appear in newborns. Up to 70% of boys with X-linked H/AED show alopecia during infancy. The ability to sweat is reduced or absent; therefore, more than 90% of children have recurrent fever spikes and 6% of children have febrile seizures during the first year of life.

By contrast, autosomal forms of H/AED are caused by mutations in the *EDAR* or *EDARADD* genes, show either a dominant or recessive inheritance, and are much less frequent than the X-linked forms. It is difficult to distinguish autosomal dominant/recessive H/AED and X-linked H/AED clinically. The similarity of clinical symptoms for these different types of H/AED is explained by the involvement of a common pathway, the NF-κB-signaling pathway.

X-linked hypohidrotic ED with immunodeficiency is an X-linked recessive disorder with a frequency of 1 per 250,000 newborns [9]. Most patients show small deletions or non-sense mutations in the zinc finger domain of *NEMO* that do not lead to a complete loss of NF-κB activation but reduce or alter the function of the NF-κB pathway [10]. Therefore, mothers of patients with X-linked H/AED with immunodeficiency have skin lesions reminiscent of IP, as well as variable manifestations of H/AED [6]. In addition, these patients suffer from serious and recurrent bacterial infections and an increased risk of inflammatory diseases.

In cases of autosomal dominant inheritance, the patients have an *IκBα* mutation that prevents the phosphorylation and degradation of the IκBα protein, resulting in abnormal activation of NF-κB. These patients have T-cell immunodeficiency, along with classic characteristics of H/AHED.

Odonto-onycho-dermal dysplasia is an autosomal recessive disorder caused by mutations in the *WNT10A* gene [11]. The *WNT* gene is involved in a signaling pathway regulating the development of ectodermally derived tissue during embryogenesis and adult life. Therefore, *WNT10A* is important for the formation or function of teeth, hair, nails, sweat glands, and lingual papillae [12, 13]. Characteristic skin lesions are telangiectatic, atrophic plaques in the face, keratosis pilaris, palmoplantar hyperkeratosis, hyperhidrosis, hypotrichosis, tooth and nail dysplasia, and a smooth tongue with reduced or absent papillae. In this case, abnormal sweating indicates hyperhidrosis, and some patients may have slight mental retardation [14–16]. The treatments for H/AED treat the symptoms only.

Incontinentia Pigmenti

IP is an X-linked dominant inherited disease caused by mutations in the *IKBKG/NEMO* gene, encoding NEMO/IKK-γ, a regulatory protein of NF-κB. IP affects the skin in all patients but also affects other ectodermal tissues such as the teeth, hair, nails, eyes, and central nervous system. Skin lesions are highly diagnostic because they appear in neonates as a repeated skin inflammation. Skin lesions of IP are divided into 4 periods, the vesiculobullous stage (up to 1–3 weeks), followed by a verrucous stage, hyperpigmented stage (12 weeks to 4 years), and finally a hypopigmented stage usually lasting the lifetime (fig. 2) [17]. The severity of the disease is related to the neurological and/or ocular impairment, of which the prevalence is approximately 30%.

Because IP is an X-linked dominant inheritance disease, it is usually lethal in males during embryogenesis. Many H/AED male patients with immune deficiency are reported to have hypomorphic *IKBKG* missense mutations [10, 18–20]. Although the causative genes are similar, H/AED with immune deficiency and IP exhibit completely different clinical symptoms. This may depend on the degree of genomic alterations and instability due to the structural architecture of the genome locus [21].

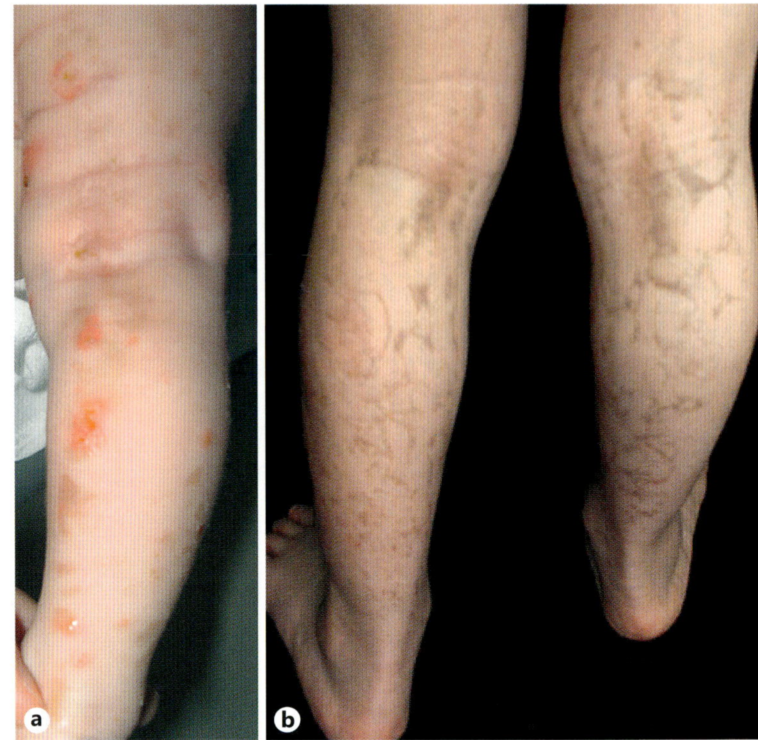

Fig. 2. Skin manifestations of IP: vesiculobullous stage (**a**) and hyperpigmented stage (**b**).

Fabry Disease

Fabry disease is an X-linked lysosomal storage disorder resulting from a deficiency of a lysosomal enzyme, α-galactosidase A, which results in the progressive accumulation of α-D-galactosyl glycosphingolipids, particularly globotriaosylceramide (Gb3), in lysosomes and disrupts the function of affected cells of the entire body.

Histopathologically, deposits of glycosphingolipids are detected using tissues stained with toluidine blue or methylene blue/azure after fixation with glutaraldehyde, which yields dark blue cytoplasmic inclusions under light microscopy. The deposits are also observed as lamellate membrane-like structures called myeloid or zebra bodies using electron microscopy. In the skin, Fabry disease primarily affects endothelial cells in the superficial dermis just below the epidermis, and Gb3 accumulates in the lysosomes of vascular endothelial cells, pericytes, eccrine gland cells, and fibroblasts.

The estimated incidence of Fabry disease ranges from 1 in 40,000 to 1 in 117,000 live male births [22]. Fabry disease is diagnosed by a low blood enzyme concentration in homozygous males and genotyping in heterozygous females. Clinically, Fabry disease is divided into three main groups based on their presentation and plasma α-galactosidase level: classical Fabry disease, heterozygous females, and the cardiac variant. Classical Fabry disease consists of patients with less than 1% of the normal plasma α-galactosidase activity and usually presents in childhood with typical clinical symptoms, including hypohidrosis. Heterozygous females are patients with 0–100% of the normal plasma α-galactosidase activity. These patients show disease manifestations from mild to severe because of the abnormal-inactivation (lyonization) ratio. The cardiac variant of Fabry disease may be an important cause of idiopathic left ventricular hypertrophy or late-onset hypertrophic cardiomyopathy.

Clinical manifestations of the disease are hypohidrosis and consequent heat intolerance, acroparesthesia, angiokeratomas (fig. 3), corneal opacities, cardiac abnormalities, such as arrhythmias and left ventricular hypertrophy, proteinuria resulting from renal insufficiency, and cerebrovascular incidents.

Infiltration of Gb3 to the pericytes and sweat glands leads to sweating abnormalities in Fabry disease. The classic symptoms of sweating are hypohidrosis and anhidrosis. These symptoms are common and early manifestations of Fabry disease, with a higher prevalence in males than females. Hypohidrosis and anhidrosis were reported in 70–93% and 17–25% of male and female patients, respectively [23]. The sweat volume in young Fabry male patients was 0.45 ± 0.46 μl/mm^2 less than that in age-matched controls [24]. The destruction of sweat glands due to the accumulation of Gb3 causes hypohidrosis/anhidrosis. Recently, hyperhidrosis, which is much less common than hypohidrosis and is more common in females compared to males, has been found in patients with Fabry disease. Therefore, it is hypothesized that abnormal sweating may result from not only the destruction of the sweat gland itself, but also from a functional abnormality in the sweating regulatory pathways, which consist of the thermal center, neurotransmitters, and innervation of the periglandular neurotransmission.

A specific therapy for Fabry disease is enzyme replacement with recombinant human α-galactosidase A. If started during the early phase of the disease, it has potential for the control of renal and cardiac disease. However, the beneficial role has not yet been defined for central nervous system and dermal symptoms.

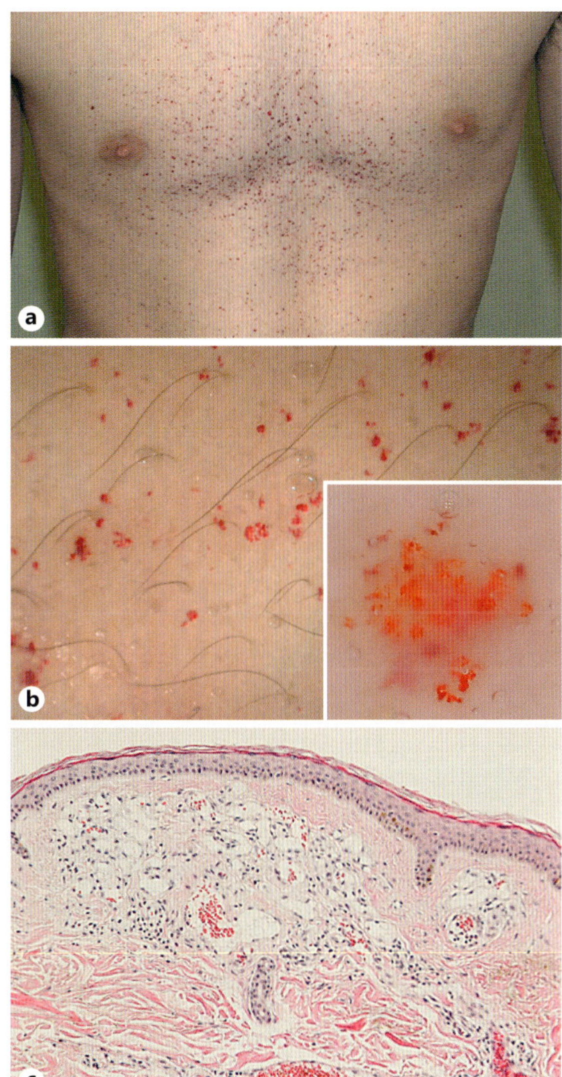

Fig. 3. Angiokeratomas in Fabry disease. **a** Angiokeratomas on the body. **b** Magnified photograph of an angiokeratoma. **c** Histopathological findings of a hematoxylin and eosin-stained angiokeratoma (original magnification ×100).

Congenital Insensitivity to Pain with Anhidrosis

CIPA is an autosomal recessive hereditary disorder characterized by generalized anhidrosis/hypohidrosis and insensitivity to pain without motor impairment [25]. CIPA is also known as hereditary sensory and autonomic neuropathy (HSAN) type IV. The incidence is estimated as 1 in 25,000 without a predilection toward sex. The incidence is higher in the Japanese, Israeli, and Bedouin populations. Although, the gene responsible for CIPA is *NTRK1* (neuropathic tyrosine kinase receptor type 1), the mechanism from which it exerts its effect is unknown. In the Japanese population, only 3 mutations, Arg554Gly frameshift (fs), Phe284Trp fs, and Asp674Tyr, account for 70% of HSAN type IV. In the Israeli and Bedouin populations, the mutation Pro621Ser fs comprises 70% of the mutations. Unlike ED or Fabry disease, the sweat glands are histologically normal. Electron microscopic examination may reveal abnormal findings of periglandular unmyelinated sweet gland motor nerve fibers.

In addition to anhidrosis/hypohidrosis and insensitivity to pain, CIPA shows neural abnormalities, such as mental retardation and cognitive impairment. Anhidrosis/hypohidrosis often causes recurrent episodes of elevated body temperature, ensuing convulsions, heat stroke, and acute encephalopathy. Insensitivity to pain also induces repeated traumas and the increased severity of the wounds, which consequently causes Charcot joint.

The causative gene of HSAN type V is *NGFB* (nerve growth factor-β), and may result in anhidrosis/hypohidrosis dominant in the extremities.

There is no specific therapy for CIPA.

References

1 Thurnam J: Two cases in which the skin, hair and teeth were imperfectly developed. Med Chir Trans 1848;31:71–82.
2 DiGiovanna JJ, Priolo M, Itin P: Approach towards a new classification for ectodermal dysplasias: integration of the clinical and molecular knowledge. Am J Med Genet A 2009;149A:2068–2070.
3 Irvine AD: Towards a unified classification of the ectodermal dysplasias: opportunities outweigh challenges. Am J Med Genet A 2009;149A:1970–1972.
4 Priolo M: Ectodermal dysplasias: an overview and update of clinical and molecular-functional mechanisms. Am J Med Genet A 2009;149A:2003–2013.
5 Garcia-Martin P, Hernandez-Martin A, Torrelo A: Ectodermal dysplasias: a clinical and molecular review. Actas Dermosifiliogr 2013;104:451–470.
6 Cluzeau C, Hadj-Rabia S, Jambou M, et al: Only four genes (EDA1, EDAR, EDARADD, and WNT10A) account for 90% of hypohidrotic/anhidrotic ectodermal dysplasia cases. Hum Mutat 2011;32: 70–72.
7 Zonana J: Hypohidrotic (anhidrotic) ectodermal dysplasia: molecular genetic research and its clinical applications. Semin Dermatol 1993;12:241–246.
8 Kere J, Srivastava AK, Montonen O, et al: X-linked anhidrotic (hypohidrotic) ectodermal dysplasia is caused by mutation in a novel transmembrane protein. Nat Genet 1996;13:409–416.
9 Orange JS, Jain A, Ballas ZK, Schneider LC, Geha RS, Bonilla FA: The presentation and natural history of immunodeficiency caused by nuclear factor kappaB essential modulator mutation. J Allergy Clin Immunol 2004;113:725–733.
10 Zonana J, Elder ME, Schneider LC, et al: A novel X-linked disorder of immune deficiency and hypohidrotic ectodermal dysplasia is allelic to incontinentia pigmenti and due to mutations in IKK-gamma (NEMO). Am J Hum Genet 2000;67:1555–1562.
11 Adaimy L, Chouery E, Megarbane H, et al: Mutation in WNT10A is associated with an autosomal recessive ectodermal dysplasia: the odonto-onycho-dermal dysplasia. Am J Hum Genet 2007;81: 821–828.
12 Nawaz S, Klar J, Wajid M, et al: WNT10A missense mutation associated with a complete odonto-onycho-dermal dysplasia syndrome. Eur J Hum Genet 2009;17:1600–1605.
13 Kantaputra P, Sripathomsawat W: WNT10A and isolated hypodontia. Am J Med Genet A 2011;155A:1119–1122.
14 Adams BB: Odonto-onycho-dermal dysplasia syndrome. J Am Acad Dermatol 2007;57:732–733.
15 Arnold WP, Merkx MA, Steijlen PM: Variant of odontoonychodermal dysplasia? Am J Med Genet 1995;59:242–244.
16 Megarbane H, Haddad M, Delague V, Renoux J, Boehm N, Megarbane A: Further delineation of the odonto-onychodermal dysplasia syndrome. Am J Med Genet A 2004;129A:193–197.
17 Landy SJ, Donnai D: Incontinentia pigmenti (Bloch-Sulzberger syndrome). J Med Genet 1993;30:53–59.
18 Bustamante J, Picard C, Boisson-Dupuis S, Abel L, Casanova JL: Genetic lessons learned from X-linked Mendelian susceptibility to mycobacterial diseases. Ann NY Acad Sci 2011;1246:92–101.

19 Picard C, Casanova JL, Puel A: Infectious diseases in patients with IRAK-4, MyD88, NEMO, or IκBα deficiency. Clin Microbiol Rev 2011;24:490–497.
20 Dupuis-Girod S, Corradini N, Hadj-Rabia S, et al: Osteopetrosis, lymphedema, anhidrotic ectodermal dysplasia, and immunodeficiency in a boy and incontinentia pigmenti in his mother. Pediatrics 2002;109:e97.
21 Fusco F, Paciolla M, Napolitano F, et al: Genomic architecture at the incontinentia pigmenti locus favours de novo pathological alleles through different mechanisms. Hum Mol Genet 2012;21:1260–1271.
22 Meikle PJ, Hopwood JJ, Clague AE, Carey WF: Prevalence of lysosomal storage disorders. JAMA 1999;281:249–254.
23 Ramaswami U, Whybra C, Parini R, et al: Clinical manifestations of Fabry disease in children: data from the Fabry Outcome Survey. Acta Paediatr 2006;95:86–92.
24 Ries M, Gupta S, Moore DF, et al: Pediatric Fabry disease. Pediatrics 2005;115:e344–e355.
25 Ravichandra KS, Kandregula CR, Koya S, Lakhotia D: Congenital insensitivity to pain and anhydrosis: diagnostic and therapeutic dilemmas revisited. Int J Clin Pediatr Dent 2015;8:75–81.

Mari Wataya-Kaneda
Department of Dermatology
Graduate School of Medicine, Osaka University
2-2 Yamadaoka, Suita-shi
Osaka 565-0871 (Japan)
E-Mail mkaneda@derma.med.osaka-u.ac.jp

Yokozeki H, Murota H, Katayama I (eds): Perspiration Research.
Curr Probl Dermatol. Basel, Karger, 2016, vol 51, pp 50–56 (DOI: 10.1159/000446758)

Histamine Modulates Sweating and Affects Clinical Manifestations of Atopic Dermatitis

Aya Takahashi • Saki Tani • Hiroyuki Murota • Ichiro Katayama
Department of Dermatology, Course of Integrated Medicine, Graduate School of Medicine, Osaka University, Osaka, Japan

Abstract

Many factors such as food or environmental allergens, bacteria, fungi, and mental stress aggravate the condition of atopic dermatitis (AD) eczema. Sweating can also exacerbate AD, and patients are aware of that. In the past, it has been reported that contamination of skin surface antigens by sweat induces acute allergic reactions and that sweating functions of AD patients via axonal reflexes are decreased. Histamine demonstrably inhibits acetylcholine-induced sweating in both mice and humans via histamine H_1 receptor-mediated signaling. In sweat glands, acetylcholine inactivates glycogen synthase kinase 3β (GSK3β), a kinase involved in endocytosis and secretion, whereas simultaneous stimulation with histamine activates GSK3β and inhibits sweat secretion. Thus, histamine might be involved in the mechanism of abnormal skin dryness in patients with AD via decreasing sweat secretion. On another front, some patients secrete sweat normally. Patients with regular sweating are prone to develop skin disorders such as papules or erythema by residual sweat left on the skin surface. Patients with decreased sweating are prone to develop disorders characterized by xerosis, lichenoid changes, prurigo by elevated skin temperature, skin dryness, and compromised skin conditions. Careful inspection of skin manifestations provides a good indication of a patient's ability to sweat.

Atopic dermatitis (AD) is an inflammatory skin disease characterized by itch and chronic relapse. AD patients present with various types of eczema, and many factors such as food or environmental allergens, bacteria, fungi, and mental stress aggravate this condition. Sweating is also thought to exacerbate AD based on the analysis of a large-scale questionnaire survey, in which patients complained about eczema becoming worse after sweating. This subjective impression sometimes misleads both patients and medical staff, causing them to avoid sweating activities. To investigate the impact of sweating on AD, questionnaires relevant to exacerbating factors were administered

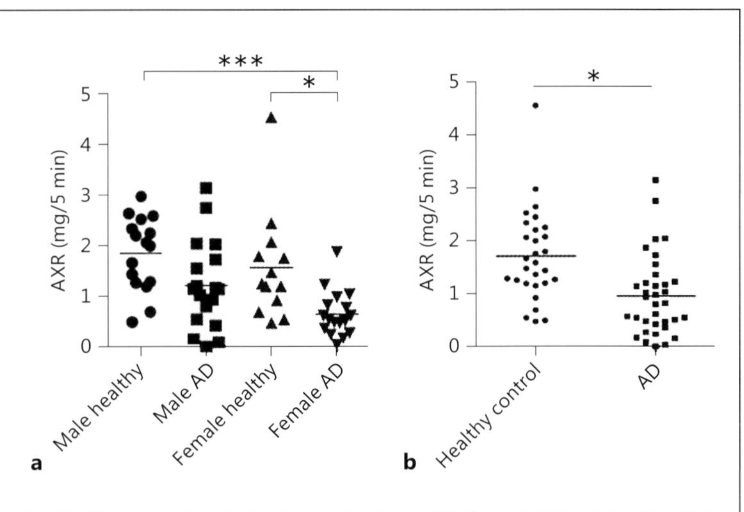

Fig. 1. Measurement results of AXR-mediated sweating in healthy and AD subjects. **a** Differences in AXR with regard to gender, measured by QSART in healthy and AD subjects. * $p < 0.05$, *** $p < 0.0005$; one-way analysis of variance, Bonferroni's multiple comparison (male healthy: n = 16, male AD: n = 18, female healthy: n = 13, female AD: n = 17). **b** Results for AXR, measured by QSART in healthy and AD subjects. * $p < 0.05$; unpaired t test (healthy: n = 38, AD: n = 35). These data are reprinted from Takahashi et al. [7].

to 66 AD patients in our hospital. Almost all of them answered that sweating is an exacerbating factor, while half of them answered that their lesioned sites do not overlap with sweaty skin. This result indicates that sweat might not play an immediate role in disease exacerbation in the latter group. Sweating is not only an exacerbating factor, but is also essential for skin health. This section describes the influence of sweating on AD and how to manage sweating effectively.

Sweating and Skin Barrier Function in Atopic Dermatitis

Several factors maintain skin homeostasis and regulate the permeability and solidity of the skin barrier. Sweating is involved in the maintenance of skin homeostasis, with antimicrobial [1, 2] and moisturizing effects [3], and in the regulation of skin surface pH [4]. In evaluating methods to assess skin barrier function in AD, many reports have examined transepidermal water loss and water-holding capacity (WHC) [5, 6]. The WHC of the skin in AD patients is lower and their transepidermal water loss is higher than those in healthy subjects because of the dysfunction of the skin barrier. In addition, an AD patient's acetylcholine (ACh)-mediated sweating activity is decreased [3, 7] (fig. 1). Abnormal skin physiology, such as decreased sweating, has also been thought to be involved in the pathogenesis of AD. It has been reported that sweat volume mediated by axonal reflexes (AXR) decreases according to the degree of psychological stress and anxiety in AD patients, as well as to their poor responsiveness to ACh [3, 8–10]. ACh-induced sweat volume can be measured by the Quantitative Sudomotor Axon Reflex Test (QSART). In this test, ACh is passed into the skin by iontophoresis, and both the amount of sweating generated by the peripheral nerve AXR and the time required before sweating starts can be measured [3, 11]. An AD patient's AXR sweat volume is about one half that of a healthy subject, and the latency time to sweat onset after ACh stimulation is significantly prolonged compared with that of a healthy subject [3, 7]. It has been reported that AXR sweat volume positively correlates with WHC in healthy subjects, but not in subjects with AD [7]. These results suggest that sweat might be a major source of water in the stratum corneum and that func-

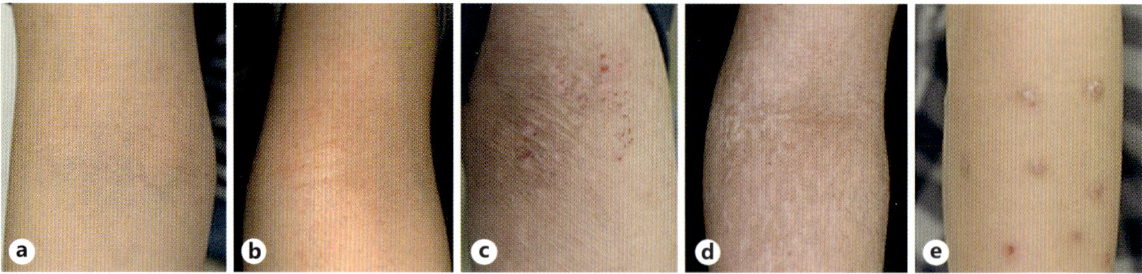

Fig. 2. Various skin manifestations of the cubital fossa in AD patients: no eruption (**a**), red papules (**b**), xerosis and scratch dermatitis (**c**), lichenoid change (**d**), and prurigo (**e**).

tional abnormalities of the stratum corneum in AD patients might impair the evaluation of WHC, even in cases of sufficient sweat volume.

Sweating Affects Manifestations of Atopic Dermatitis

Several types of eczema, such as red papules, xerosis, xerotic eczema, miliaria, lichenoid changes, and prurigo, are observed in patients with AD (fig. 2). In particular, eczema on the cubital or popliteal fossa is frequently observed in many AD patients [12–14]. Although this is our subjective impression in daily clinical practice, many adult cases of AD with prolonged clinical courses develop eruptions that avoid the cubital fossa. It has been revealed that AXR sweat volume correlates with clinical manifestations of the cubital fossa in subjects with AD [7]. In that study, 73 AD patients were divided into two groups, those with above- or below-average AXR sweat volume in the cubital fossa, and their clinical features at the same sites were assessed. Compared with the above-average sweating group (more than the average AXR), the below-average sweating group was associated with a much higher incidence of clinical manifestations, such as lichenoid eczema, prurigo, or papules (table 1). However, the above-average sweating group tended to have no eruptions. As shown in previous reports, AD may induce a hypohidrosis condition, and it is conceivable that sweating occurs only sparsely. Then why do AD patients think that sweating is an exacerbating factor for AD? We speculate that sweating can induce pruritus and exacerbate symptoms via elevated skin temperature due to hypohidrosis. Furthermore, hypohidrosis is involved in skin dryness and increased susceptibility to infection.

Histamine as a Factor to Reduce Sweating Ability

Impact of Histamine on Sweat Secretion

In AD, two mechanisms are believed to reduce sweating ability. One is an abnormal excretion of sweat to the skin surface. The mechanism is considered to be either occlusion associated with the formation of keratotic plugs in sweat pores [15] or leakage of sweat from sweat ducts into surrounding tissues [16]. Another mechanism is an abnormal production and secretion of sweat by sweat glands, reportedly via an autonomic imbalance or decrease in the response to ACh [17]. In past reports, histamine has been shown to impair the excretion of sweat. The histamine receptor, a 7-transmembrane receptor, has a similar structure to that of the ACh receptor [18]. A recent

Table 1. Frequency of characteristic clinical manifestations in below- or above-average sweating subjects with AD

	Lichenoid eczema	Papules, prurigo	No eczematous change	Total
Above-average sweating[1]	6 (23.1)	5 (23.8)	10 (83.8)	21 (35.6)
Below-average sweating[2]	20 (76.9)	16 (76.2)	2 (16.7)	38 (64.4)
Total	26 (100)	21 (100)	12 (100)	59 (100)

Figures in parentheses are percentages. Pearson's χ^2 test for independence, $p = 0.0001$. This table was reprinted from Takahashi et al. [7] with permission of the Japanese Association of Allergology. [1] Above the average of AXR-mediated sweating volume. [2] Below the average of AXR-mediated sweating volume.

study showed that histamine suppresses ACh-induced sweating [19, 20]. These inhibitory effects of histamine on ACh-mediated sweating in humans were assessed by QSART (fig. 3). When histamine was iontophoretically applied with ACh simultaneously, QSART-measured results were significantly decreased compared with results from stimulation solely by Ach [19].

Sweat glands express histamine receptors [H_1 receptor (H_1R), H_2R, and H_4R] and the muscarinic 3 receptor (M_3R). ACh receptors in mouse eccrine sweat glands are predominantly type M_3R [21]. Protein gene product 9.5-positive peripheral nerve fibers costain with antibodies against H_1R, H_2R, and M_3R, but myoepithelial cells do not stain with antibodies against H_1R, H_2R, H_4R, and M_3R [19]. As the histamine-mediated inhibition of sweat secretion is abrogated by the administration of an H_1R antagonist, an H_1R-mediated signal plays prominently in this phenomenon. These results suggest that there might be cross-talk between two distinct pathways downstream of H_1R and ACh receptors in sweat glands.

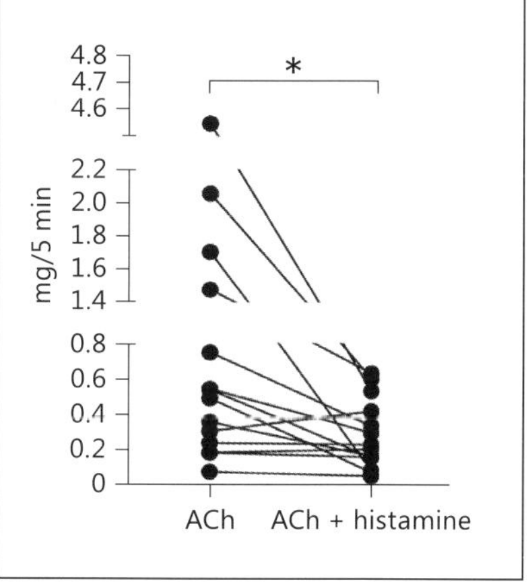

Fig. 3. Histamine reduces AXR sweat volume in humans. Effects of simultaneous administration of histamine on results of a quantitative sudomotor AXR test was assessed in the same individual (n = 13). * $p < 0.05$; paired t test. These data are reprinted from Matsui et al. [19] with the publisher's permission.

Histamine Blocks Phosphorylation of Glycogen Synthase Kinase 3β Activated by ACh Stimulation

Glycogen synthase kinase 3 (GSK3) is a serine-threonine kinase that exists as two isoforms, α and β [22]. GSK3 was originally identified as an inhibitor of glycogen synthase [23], and it contributes to various phenomena such as glycogen metabolism, cell cycle progression, cell proliferation and differentiation, cell membrane transport, and permeability [24–28]. Boini et al. [29] showed that GSK3β is involved in the glomerular

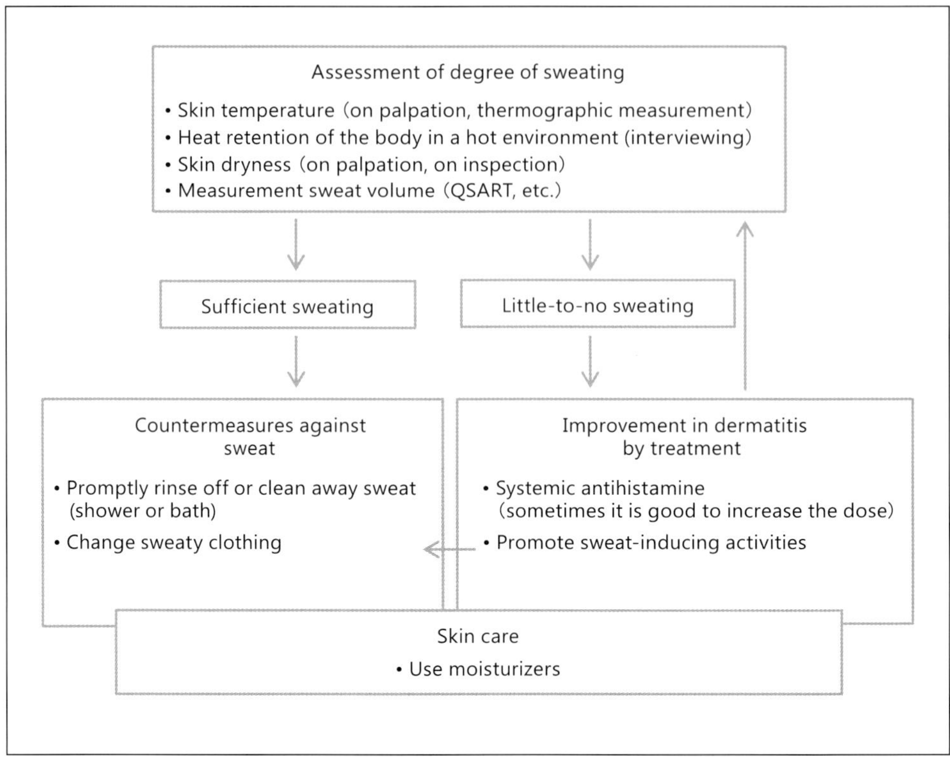

Fig. 4. Flow chart for managing sweat in patients with AD.

filtration function of the kidney. Sweat glands are also filters in the skin, so the idea that GSK3β might be involved in sweat secretion as well as glomerular filtration was suggested. A phosphorylation antibody array using whole-skin lysates found that GSK3α/β was phosphorylated by ACh alone, but not by either ACh plus histamine or histamine alone. Immunohistochemical staining of skin sections confirmed that phosphorylation of GSK3β was observed in sweat glands of ACh-treated skin, but not in Ach- and histamine-treated skin [19]. From these results, it is conceivable that histamine inhibits the secretion of sweat from sweat glands by suppressing the ACh signal upstream of GSK3β.

Sweat Allergy

The frequency of positive reactions in skin testing to autologous sweat among AD patients was significantly higher than healthy subjects [30, 31]. Moreover, many patients with AD exhibit a positive result in histamine-release tests for sweat antigens; this reaction has been referred to as 'sweat allergy' [32, 33]. In practice, this positive test response is not the result of an allergy to sweat itself, as the responses were confirmed to be due to *Malassezia globosa*-derived antigens (MGL_1304) admixed with sweat-derived proteins [34]. Various skin surface antigens that are in sweat might be involved in immediate allergic reactions. For a detailed discussion of the mechanism involved in sweat allergy, see the chapter by Hiragun and Hide et al. [this vol., pp. 101–108].

Managing Sweat in Patients with Atopic Dermatitis

To manage abnormal sweating ability in AD patients, the following points should be kept in mind. (1) Although the skin hydration level correlates with sweat volume in healthy subjects, it does not reflect sweat volume in AD patients due to the decreased WHC of the stratum corneum. (2) The amount of AXR sweat in AD patients is about one half the levels in healthy individuals. Additionally, a prolonged latent time until sweating following the administration of ACh was found in AD patients compared with healthy subjects. (3) Histamine inhibits excretion of sweat from sweat glands. (4) Various skin surface antigens, which contaminate sweat, might be involved in immediate allergic reactions and exacerbate AD symptoms.

With these points in mind, dermatologists can provide guidance to patients for managing sweat (fig. 4). First, patients should not avoid sweating, but should be given opportunities to sweat. It should be noted that AD patients cannot sweat enough. Thus, patients should be advised to start sweating in small steps. When patients sweat sufficiently, it is better to advise them to change out of their sweaty clothes and promptly rinse off, shower, or wipe off with a wet towel. Showering is an effective measure after sweating [35–37]. These measures are intended to avoid causing either irritation to the skin or alterations in the skin's bacterial flora. To increase the positive effects of sweating, guidance to restore the impaired WHC of the stratum corneum by applying moisturizers can be helpful for patients.

References

1 Rieg S, Steffen H, Seeber S, Humeny A, Kalbacher H, Dietz K, Garbe C, Schittek B: Deficiency of dermcidin-derived antimicrobial peptides in sweat of patients with atopic dermatitis correlates with an impaired innate defense of human skin in vivo. J Immunol 2005;174:8003–8010.

2 Schittek B, Paulmann M, Senyürek I, Steffen H: The role of antimicrobial peptides in human skin and in skin infectious diseases. Infect Disord Drug Targets 2008;8:135–143.

3 Eishi K, Lee JB, Bae SJ, Takenaka M, Katayama I: Impaired sweating function in adult atopic dermatitis: results of the quantitative sudomotor axon reflex test. Br J Dermatol 2002;147:683–688.

4 Schmid-Wendtner MH, Korting HC: The pH of the skin surface and its impact on the barrier function. Skin Pharmacol Physiol 2006;19:296–302.

5 Thune P, Nilsen T, Hanstad IK, Gustavsen T, Lovig Dahl H: The water barrier function of the skin in relation to the water content of stratum corneum, pH and skin lipids. The effect of alkaline soap and syndet on dry skin in elderly, non-atopic patients. Acta Derm Venereol 1988;68:277–283.

6 Werner Y, Lindberg M: Transepidermal water loss in dry and clinically normal skin in patients with atopic dermatitis. Acta Derm Venereol 1985;65:102–105.

7 Takahashi A, Murota H, Matsui S, Kijima A, Kitaba S, Lee JB, Katayama I: Decreased sudomotor function is involved in the formation of atopic eczema in the cubital fossa. Allergol Int 2013;62:473–478.

8 Kijima A, Murota H, Matsui S, Takahashi A, Kimura A, Kitaba S, Lee JB, Katayama I: Abnormal axon reflex-mediated sweating correlates with high state of anxiety in atopic dermatitis. Allergol Int 2012;61:469–473.

9 Kitaba S, Matsui S, Iimuro E, Nishioka M, Kijima A, Umegaki N, Murota H, Katayama I: Four cases of atopic dermatitis complicated by Sjogren's syndrome: link between dry skin and autoimmune anhidrosis. Allergol Int 2011;60:387–391.

10 Katayama I, Bae SJ, Hamasaki Y, Igawa K, Miyazaki Y, Yokozeki H, Nishioka K: Stress response, tachykinin, and cutaneous inflammation. J Investig Dermatol Symp Proc 2001;6:81–86.

11 Low PA, Caskey PE, Tuck RR, Fealey RD, Dyck PJ: Quantitative sudomotor axon reflex test in normal and neuropathic subjects. Ann Neurol 1983;14:573–580.

12 Jepsen KF, Flyvholm MA: Identification of subjects with atopic dermatitis in questionnaire studies. Contact Dermatitis 2007;56:218–223.

13 Benn CS, Benfeldt E, Andersen PK, Olesen AB, Melbye M, Bjorksten B: Atopic dermatitis in young children: diagnostic criteria for use in epidemiological studies based on telephone interviews. Acta Derm Venereol 2003;83:347–350.

14 Nnoruka EN: Current epidemiology of atopic dermatitis in south-eastern Nigeria. Int J Dermatol 2004;43:739–744.

15 Papa CM, Kligman AM: Mechanisms of eccrine anidrosis. I. High level blockade. J Invest Dermatol 1966;47:1–9.

16 Shiohara T, Doi T, Hayakawa J: Defective sweating responses in atopic dermatitis. Curr Probl Dermatol 2011;41:68–79.

17 Greene RM, Winkelmann RK, Opfer-Gehrking TL, Low PA: Sweating patterns in atopic dermatitis patients. Arch Dermatol Res 1989;281:373–376.

18 Kitaba S, Matsui S, Iimuro E, Nishioka M, Kijima A, Umegaki N, Murota H, Katayama I: Four cases of atopic dermatitis complicated by Sjogren's syndrome: link between dry skin and autoimmune anhidrosis. Allergol Int 2011;60:387–391.
19 Matsui S, Murota H, Takahashi A, Yang L, Lee JB, Omiya K, Ohmi M, Kikuta J, Ishii M, Katayama I: Dynamic analysis of histamine-mediated attenuation of acetylcholine-induced sweating via GSK3β activation. J Invest Dermatol 2014;134:326–334.
20 Matsui S, Murota H, Ono E, Kikuta J, Ishii M, Katayama I: Olopatadine hydrochloride restores histamine-induced impaired sweating. J Dermatol Sci 2014;74:260–261.
21 Vilches JJ, Navarro X, Verdu E: Functional sudomotor responses to cholinergic agonists and antagonists in the mouse. J Auton Nerv Syst 1995;55:105–111.
22 Woodgett JR: Molecular cloning and expression of glycogen synthase kinase-3/factor A. EMBO J 1990;9:2431–2438.
23 Buschiazzo A, Ugalde JE, Guerin ME, Shepard W, Ugalde RA, Alzari PM: Crystal structure of glycogen synthase: homologous enzymes catalyze glycogen synthesis and degradation. EMBO J 2004;23:3196–3205.
24 Doble BW, Woodgett JR: GSK-3: tricks of the trade for a multi-tasking kinase. J Cell Sci 2003;116:1175–1186.
25 Jope RS, Johnson GV: The glamour and gloom of glycogen synthase kinase-3. Trends Biochem Sci 2004;29:95–102.
26 Wang H, Brown J, Martin M: Glycogen synthase kinase 3: a point of convergence for the host inflammatory response. Cytokine 2011;53:130–140.
27 Adachi A, Kano F, Saido TC, Murata M: Visual screening and analysis for kinase-regulated membrane trafficking pathways that are involved in extensive beta-amyloid secretion. Genes Cells 2009;14:355–369.
28 Rexhepaj R, Dërmaku-Sopjani M, Gehring EM, Sopjani M, Kempe DS, Föller M, Lang F: Stimulation of electrogenic glucose transport by glycogen synthase kinase 3. Cell Physiol Biochem 2010;26:641–646.
29 Boini KM, Amann K, Kempe D, Alessi DR, Lang F: Proteinuria in mice expressing PKB/SGK-resistant GSK3. Am J Physiol Renal Physiol 2009;296:F153–F159.
30 Adachi K, Aoki T: IgE antibody to sweat in atopic dermatitis. Acta Derm Venereol Suppl (Stockh) 1989;144:83–87.
31 Hide M, Tanaka T, Yamamura Y, Koro O, Yamamoto S: IgE-mediated hypersensitivity against human sweat antigen in patients with atopic dermatitis. Acta Derm Venereol 2002;82:335–340.
32 Tanaka A, Tanaka T, Suzuki H, Ishii K, Kameyoshi Y, Hide M: Semi-purification of the immunoglobulin E-sweat antigen acting on mast cells and basophils in atopic dermatitis. Exp Dermatol 2006;15:283–290.
33 Takahagi S, Tanaka T, Ishii K, Suzuki H, Kameyoshi Y, Shindo H, Hide M: Sweat antigen induces histamine release from basophils of patients with cholinergic urticarial associated with atopic dermatitis. Br J Dermatol 2009;160:426–428.
34 Hiragun T, Ishii K, Hiragun M, Suzuki H, Kan T, Mihara S, Yanase Y, Bartels J, Schröder JM, Hide M: Fungal protein MGL_1304 in sweat is an allergen for atopic dermatitis patients. J Allergy Clin Immunol 2013;132:608–615.
35 Kameyoshi Y, Tanaka T, Mochizuki M, Koro O, Mihara S, Hiragun T, Tanaka M, Hide M: Taking showers at school is beneficial for children with severer atopic dermatitis (in Japanese). Arerugi 2008;57:130–137.
36 Mochizuki H, Muramatsu R, Tadaki H, Mizuno T, Arakawa H, Morikawa A: Effects of skin care with shower therapy on children with atopic dermatitis in elementary schools. Pediatr Dermatol 2009;26:223–225.
37 Murota H, Takahashi A, Nishioka M, Matsui S, Terao M, Kitaba S, Katayama I: Showering reduces atopic dermatitis in elementary school students. Eur J Dermatol 2010;20:410–411.

Aya Takahashi
Department of Dermatology
Course of Integrated Medicine
Graduate School of Medicine
Osaka University
2-2 Yamadaoka, Suita-shi
Osaka 565-0871 (Japan)
E-Mail aya529@green.ocn.ne.jp

Yokozeki H, Murota H, Katayama I (eds): Perspiration Research.
Curr Probl Dermatol. Basel, Karger, 2016, vol 51, pp 57–61 (DOI: 10.1159/000446760)

Sweating in Systemic Abnormalities: Uremia and Diabetes Mellitus

Hiroyuki Murota
Department of Dermatology, Course of Integrated Medicine, Graduate School of Medicine, Osaka University, Osaka, Japan

Abstract
Sweating disorders are sometimes observed in various systemic diseases that include genetic disorders, organ damage, metabolic impairment, autoimmune diseases, and neuropathic disorders. In these diseases, various symptoms such as autonomic failures, psychopathic disorders, abnormal skin innervation, and sweat gland dysfunction can interact with one another in diverse ways, resulting in impaired sweating. This review focuses on the influence of uremia (with or without hemodialysis) and diabetes mellitus on impaired sweating. Dialysis patients perspire less, but their sweat contains higher levels of uremic toxins than do healthy subjects. Neuropathic disorders in diabetes patients develop in relation to disease severity and can impair sweating. Physicians should consider the development of various problems, such as increased body temperature, dry skin, and increased susceptibility to infection, due to decreased sweating, as they are often found in these systemic abnormalities.

Hypohidrosis is frequently found in association with local and systemic disorders [1, 2]. The background diseases associated with decreased sweating can be divided into three major groups [2]: (1) external factors such as drugs and somatic factors, (2) congenital or acquired anomalies associated with skin disease, and (3) neurogenic causes associated with central or peripheral nervous abnormalities. Drugs that can result in hypohidrosis may be prescribed for anticholinergic effects, nerve-impairing effects (e.g. botulinum toxin), modulation of body temperature regulation (e.g. opioid agents and α-receptor antagonist/agonist drugs), and necrosis of sweat glands (e.g. barbiturates) [2]. Somatic factors, such as posttraumatic sequelae (e.g. burn, radiation exposure, and surgical scars), can cause local hypohidrosis. Some skin diseases can also cause secondary hypohidrosis. Fabry disease, hypohidrotic ectodermal dysplasia, and pigment incontinence are representative congenital skin diseases that develop hypohidrosis. The acquired skin diseases that ex-

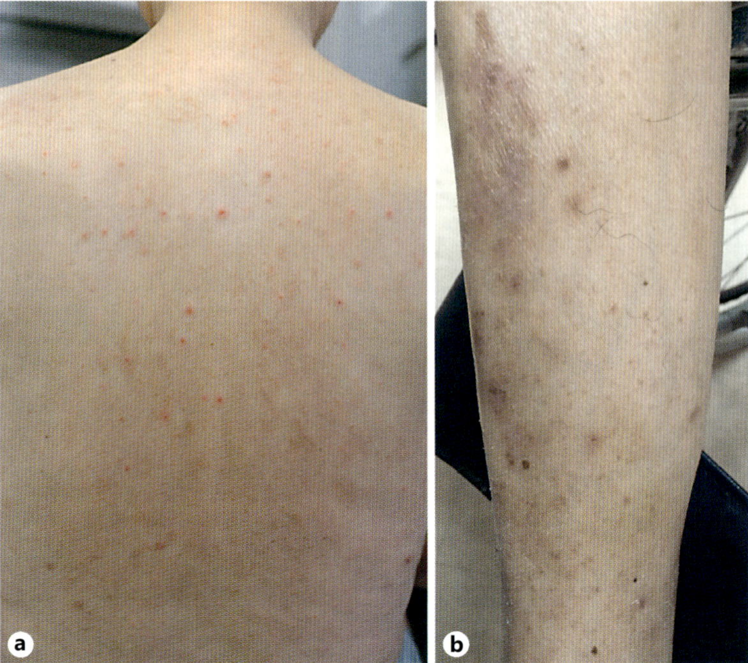

Fig. 1. Clinical manifestation of dry skin observed in diabetic and uremic subjects. **a** Abnormal dryness of back skin accompanied by prurigo observed in a subject with diabetes mellitus. **b** Dryness, pruritus, and pigmentation of lower leg skin observed in a uremic patient undergoing hemodialysis.

hibit hypohidrosis include atopic dermatitis, cholinergic urticaria, Sjögren's syndrome, systemic scleroderma, and graft-versus-host disease, all of which cause atrophy of the sweat glands [2, 3]. The pathogenic mechanism of cholinergic urticaria is not currently clear, though some reports suggest its pathogenesis is due to decreased expression of acetylcholine receptors or acetylcholine esterase [4, 5]. Reduced sweating has been identified in atopic dermatitis [6, 7], and the mechanism has been partially elucidated (the mechanism is described in detail in the chapter by Takahashi et al. [this vol., pp. 50–56]).

Some neurological disorders can result in hypohidrosis [2]. Central nervous disorders (e.g. cerebrovascular disease, encephalitis, cervical myelopathy, multiple system atrophy, tumors, and multiple sclerosis) and peripheral nervous disorders (e.g. diabetes, neuropathies associated with alcohol addiction, demyelinating polyneuropathy, and autonomic neuropathy) are referred to as representative nervous disorders. Thus, certain events, such as inhibition of acetylcholine action, organic disorders of the sweat glands, body temperature dysregulation, or neurological abnormalities can be a cause of hypohidrosis [2].

Diabetes Mellitus and Sweating

Diabetes mellitus is usually associated with various systemic complications, such as metabolic, cardiovascular, and nervous anomalies. The pathophysiological diagnosis of this disease promotes awareness that diabetes mellitus may interfere with a patient's thermoregulation and skin homeostasis via dysregulation of peripheral blood flow and sweating (fig. 1a). Patients with diabetes show low levels of adaptability to changes in environmental temperatures due to decreased vasoconstriction responses. Low blood glucose levels and diabetic ketoacidosis may cause hypothermia and can result in decreased sweating [8]. Diabetic neuropathy, as characterized by autonomic nervous dysfunction, involves the development of dysesthesia, protracted wound healing, and unusual modulation of skin homeostasis [9]. Thus, physiological and pathological skin function testing can yield valuable information for understanding the severity of impaired autonomic functions [10].

Thermoregulatory sweat testing in diabetic subjects involving the measurement of myogram and quantitative sudomotor axon reflexes indicates that anhidrosis areas spread extensively [11]. Sweat glands receive sympathetic innervation, and the loss of sympathetic nerve fiber density is found in diabetic sweat glands in correlation with glycemic control [12].

In the assessment presented here, skin samples from the lower legs were immunohistologically stained with protein gene product 9.5, a general neuronal marker, and the sweat gland innervation index (SGII) was calculated [SGII = (nerve fiber area/sweat gland area) × 100%]. SGII correlates with the measurement of functional sweating and HbA_{1C}-levels. However, when we evaluate SGII, we should take heed of age- and sex-related differences in sudomotor functions and should consider the calculated score carefully.

On another front, glucose is a component of sweat [13]. Transient elevation of glucose concentrations in sweat [up to 0.6–1.2 mg/dl (normal range: 0.2–0.5 mg/dl)] was found concurrently with elevation of blood glucose levels [up to 200–250 mg/dl (normal 80 mg/dl)] [14, 15]. Thus, great expectations are being placed on glucose levels in sweat to formulate noninvasive methods for determining blood glucose levels.

Uremia and Sweating

As there are structural similarities between kidney tubules and sweat glands, detailed assessments of sweat have been conducted in uremic patients. Yosipovitch et al. [16] measured and compared the electrolyte content of sweat derived from uremic patients and healthy subjects. Uremic patients showed predominately decreased sweating and high potassium levels in sweat compared to healthy subjects. Calcium levels in sweat were negatively correlated to sweat volumes. These results indicate that sweating may have a compensatory role for renal failure. Another study evaluated the serum concentrations of several hormones that regulate electrolyte concentrations in the sweat of uremic patients under hot conditions [17]. Baseline blood levels of plasma renin activity, aldosterone, vasopressin, and atrial natriuretic peptide were higher in uremic patients than in healthy subjects. After exposing subjects to hot conditions, significant increases in levels of plasma renin activity, aldosterone, and vasopressin were found in both uremic patients and healthy subjects, indicating that altered hormonal regulation did not explain the abnormal sweating in uremic patients. The pathological abnormalities of the sweat glands in uremic patients remain to be identified. On the contrary, another report found that increased sweating was a common finding in uremic patients and was relieved following renal transplantation [18]. The contradicting observations about the degree of sweating in uremic patients should be clarified via comprehensive and quantitative assessment of sweat in the future.

Hemodialysis is currently the best therapy for uremia. Although dry and itchy skin as well as hypohidrosis have been observed in hemodialysis subjects (fig. 1b), the influence of hemodialysis on sweating remains controversial. Decreased sweating has been found in uremic subjects undergoing hemodialysis (fig. 2) [19]. However, another study found no difference in sweating between uremia subjects with and without hemodialysis [16]. Furthermore, measurement of skin impedance, which indicates the content of water (e.g. sweat) held on skin, after pilocarpine-treatment indicated no difference between subjects on he-

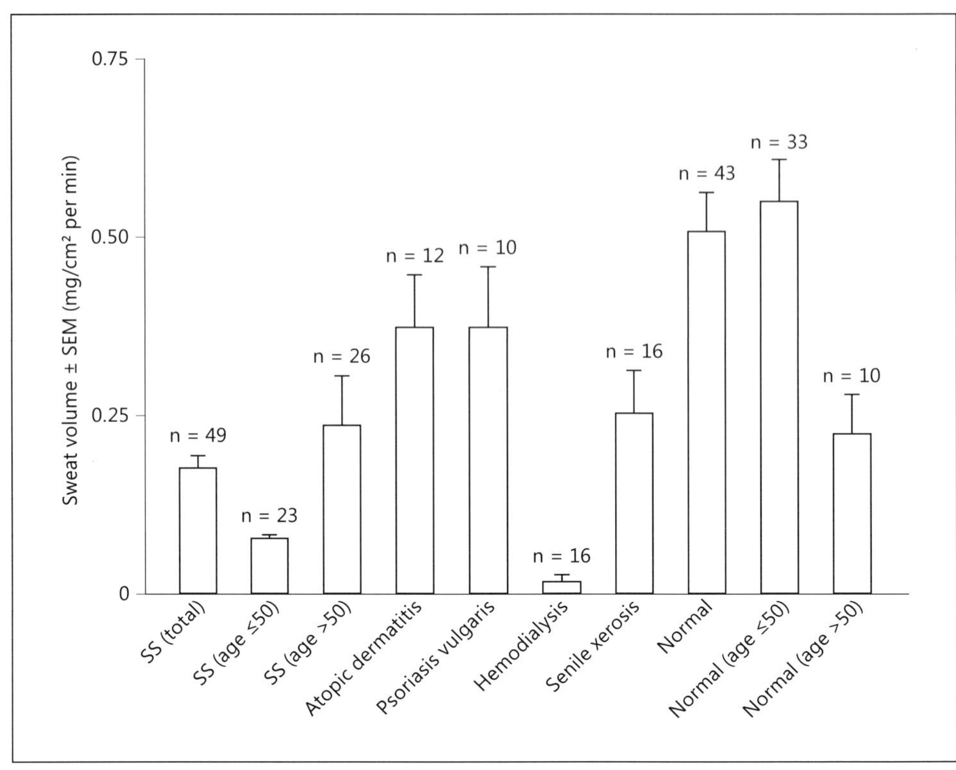

Fig. 2. Sweat volume in various skin diseases characterized by dry skin. Patients were asked to clench their hand while sweat on the surface of the hand was monitored. Sweat volume was measured by a perspirometer (Kenz-Perspiro OSS-100; Suzuken Co. Ltd., Nagoya, Japan). SS = Sjögren's syndrome. This figure was reprinted from Katayama et al. [19] with the permission of the publisher (John Wiley and Sons).

modialysis and healthy controls [20]. More precise and quantitative measurements of sweating in hemodialysis patients are required to reach a consensus. Some histopathological reports have indicated that a common feature in skin samples from hemodialysis patients is microvasculopathy. These abnormal findings become more prominent as the duration of dialysis increases. Microvessels surrounding sweat glands are important for the excretion and reabsorption of sweat. It is assumed that vascular damage in skin will greatly impair sweating. Thus, sweat-mediated excretion of various factors seems to be affected by hemodialysis in diverse ways. The level of creatinine, urea, urinary acid, uremic toxins, chloride, and sulfate are the major factors found to be increased in both blood and sweat derived from uremic patients [21–23]. Sweat and blood concentrations of these factors decreased following hemodialysis [21]. This finding could be corroborating evidence for availability of sweating as an alternative to renal failure.

References

1 Murota H, Matsui S, Ono E, Kijima A, Kikuta J, Ishii M, Katayama I: Sweat, the driving force behind normal skin: an emerging perspective on functional biology and regulatory mechanisms. J Dermatol Sci 2015;77:3–10.

2 Chia KY, Tey HL: Approach to hypohidrosis. J Eur Acad Dermatol Venereol 2013;27:799–804.

3 Katayama I, Yokozeki H, Nishioka K: Impaired sweating as an exocrine manifestation in Sjogren's syndrome. Br J Dermatol 1995;133:716–720.

4 Sawada Y, Nakamura M, Bito T, Fukamachi S, Kabashima R, Sugita K, et al: Cholinergic urticaria: studies on the muscarinic cholinergic receptor M3 in anhidrotic and hypohidrotic skin. J Invest Dermatol 2010;130:2683–2686.

5 Sawada Y, Nakamura M, Bito T, Sakabe J, Kabashima-Kubo R, Hino R, et al: Decreased expression of acetylcholine esterase in cholinergic urticaria with hypohidrosis or anhidrosis. J Invest Dermatol 2014;134:276–279.

6 Takahashi A, Murota H, Matsui S, Kijima A, Kitaba S, Lee JB, et al: Decreased sudomotor function is involved in the formation of atopic eczema in the cubital fossa. Allergol Int 2013;62:473–478.

7 Kijima A, Murota H, Matsui S, Takahashi A, Kimura A, Kitaba S, et al: Abnormal axon reflex-mediated sweating correlates with high state of anxiety in atopic dermatitis. Allergol Int 2012;61: 469–473.

8 Scott AR, Bennett T, Macdonald IA: Diabetes mellitus and thermoregulation. Can J Physiol Pharmacol 1987;65:1365–1376.

9 Tesfaye S, Boulton AJ, Dyck PJ, et al: Diabetic neuropathies: update on definitions, diagnostic criteria, estimation of severity, and treatments. Diabetes Care 2010;33:2285–2293.

10 Emanuele NV, Emanuele MA: Diabetic neuropathy: therapies for peripheral and autonomic symptoms. Geriatrics 1997; 52:40–42, 45–49.

11 Fealey RD, Low PA, Thomas JE: Thermoregulatory sweating abnormalities in diabetes mellitus. Mayo Clin Proc 1989; 64:617–628.

12 Luo KR, Chao CC, Hsieh PC, Lue JH, Hsieh ST: Effect of glycemic control on sudomotor denervation in type 2 diabetes. Diabetes Care 2012;35:612–616.

13 Boysen TS, Yanagawa Sato F, Sato K: A modified anaerobic method of sweat collection. J Appl Physiol 1984;56:1302–1307.

14 Sato K, Kang WH, Saga K, Sato KT: Biology of sweat glands and their disorders. I. Normal sweat gland function. J Am Acad Dermatol 1989;20:537–563.

15 Moyer J, Wilson D, Finkelshtein I, Wong B, Potts R: Correlation between sweat glucose and blood glucose in subjects with diabetes. Diabetes Technol Ther 2012;14:398–402.

16 Yosipovitch G, Reis J, Tur E, Blau H, Harell D, Morduchowicz G, Boner G: Sweat electrolytes in patients with advanced renal failure. J Lab Clin Med 1994;124:808–812.

17 Grzeszczak W, Kokot F, Zukowska-Szczechowska E, Woch W, Wiecek A: Influence of thermal dehydration on blood values of hormones which regulate volume and composition of electrolytes in sweat of patients with ic renal failure treated with hemodialysis (in Polish). Pol Arch Med Wewn 1991;86:346–354.

18 Altmeyer P, Kachel HG, Schäfer G, Fassbinder W: Normalization of uremic skin changes following kidney transplantation (in German). Hautarzt 1986;37: 217–221.

19 Katayama I, Yokozeki H, Nishioka K: Impaired sweating as an exocrine manifestation in Sjögren's syndrome. Br J Dermatol 1995;133:716–720.

20 Marczewski K, Janicka L, Cudny J: The effect of pilocarpine on electrodermal resistance in chronic hemodialyzed patients. Clin Nephrol 1993;39:88–91.

21 Cole DE, Boucher MJ: Increased sweat sulfate concentrations in chronic renal failure. Nephron 1986;44:92–95.

22 Sassa T, Matsuno H, Niwa M, Kozawa O, Takeda N, Niwa T, Kumada T, Uematsu T: Measurement of furancarboxylic acid, a candidate for uremic toxin, in human serum, hair, and sweat, and analysis of pharmacological actions in vitro. Arch Toxicol 2000;73:649–654.

23 al-Tamer YY, Hadi EA, al-Badrani II: Sweat urea, uric acid and creatinine concentrations in uraemic patients. Urol Res 1997;25:337–340.

Hiroyuki Murota
Department of Dermatology
Course of Integrated Medicine
Graduate School of Medicine
Osaka University
2-2 Yamadaoka, Suita-shi
Osaka, 565-0871 (Japan)
E-Mail h-murota@derma.med.osaka-u.ac.jp

Yokozeki H, Murota H, Katayama I (eds): Perspiration Research.
Curr Probl Dermatol. Basel, Karger, 2016, vol 51, pp 62–74 (DOI: 10.1159/000446780)

Abberant Sudomotor Functions in Sjögren's Syndrome: Comparable Study with Atopic Dermatitis on Dry Skin Manifestation

Ichiro Katayama

Department of Dermatology, Course of Integrated Medicine, Graduate School of Medicine, Osaka University, Osaka, Japan

Abstract

This chapter summarizes recent advances in the pathogenesis and management of Sjögren's syndrome (SS). Major topics are newly described pathomechanisms and cutaneous manifestations of SS, with special references to hypohidrosis and related mucocutaneous manifestations. Although the significance of cutaneous manifestations in SS has been gradually recognized in rheumatologists, sudomotor function has not been fully evaluated and recognized in the diagnosis of SS except by dermatologists. SS is a relatively underestimated collagen disease in contrast to systemic lupus erythematosus, systemic sclerosis, or dermatomyositis, and special care is needed not to misdiagnose SS when we see patients with common skin diseases such as drug eruption, infectious skin disease, or xerosis in daily practice. In contrast to SS, the reduced sweating function seen in atopic dermatitis (AD) is restricted only to axon reflex-induced indirect sweating, which is usually restored to normal levels after improvement of the dermatitis. Therefore, the xerotic skin lesions seen in SS and AD might be attributable to different pathomechanisms with similar dry skin manifestations. It is well known that dry skin is occasionally seen in SS, and clinical use of muscarinic M_3-receptor agonists occasionally improves this condition through recovery of sweating function. Therefore, this M_3-receptor agonist might be a promising drug and should be evaluated for the treatment of impaired sweating in AD complicated with or without SS.

Sjögren's syndrome (SS) was first reported by Henrik Sjögren, a Swedish ophthalmologist, in 1930 as a case of keratoconjunctivitis sicca associated with rheumatoid arthritis. Since then, clinical, etiological, and epidemiological analyses have been conducted throughout the world and SS is now recognized as autoimmune epithelitis or autoimmune sialadenitis induced by autoreactive T cells or tissue-specific autoantibodies. SS patients develop various types of exocrine manifestations such as autoimmune thyroiditis, interstitial nephritis, or pneumonitis during the clinical course. B-cell lymphoma/pseudolymphoma and several types of skin diseases are known as extraglandular manifestations of SS.

Known mucocutaneous manifestations associated with SS include hypohidrosis-related skin dryness and blepharitis or angular cheilitis as glandular manifestations, and hypergammaglobulinemic purpura or urticarial vasculitis as extraglandular manifestations. In addition to these skin lesions, we have previously reported that Japanese SS patients occasionally develop annular erythema (AE) with perivascular and periappendageal lymphocytic infiltration, which is characterized by a wide elevated border and central pallor [1, 2]. As only a few cases of AE in SS have been reported in Caucasians [3, 4], and because AE in Japanese SS patients shares many features with subacute cutaneous lupus erythematosus, the most photosensitive type of lupus erythematosus [5], SS manifesting with AE has been thought to be the Oriental counterpart of subacute cutaneous lupus erythematosus. However, there are substantial differences in clinical and histopathological features between the two types of skin lesions. Therefore, differentiation of SS from subacute cutaneous lupus erythematosus/systemic lupus erythematosus and significance of diversified skin manifestations seen in SS patients are important issues that need to be solved.

Although the significance of cutaneous manifestations in SS have been gradually recognized by rheumatologists as described above, sudomotor function has not been fully evaluated and recognized in the diagnosis of SS except by dermatologists.

Diagnosis of Sjögren's Syndrome

Diagnostic criteria has been proposed by several research groups from different countries. In 1993, Vitali et al. [6] proposed preliminary criteria for the classification of SS that takes 4 different classifications into consideration (Copenhagen, Greece, Japan, and California). Since then, this classification has been preferentially used for the diagnosis of SS in the world and was revised in 2002 [7]. In 1999, a Japanese research group also proposed revised Japanese criteria for SS [8]. This criteria adopted positive anti-SSA/SSB antibodies and a new diagnostic procedure to evaluate oral and ocular dryness following the 1993 classification by Vitali et al. [6], except omission of sicca components. Common items in these criteria include subjective oral and ocular symptoms and an objective laboratory test shown (table 1): dry eye (item I) and dry mouth (item II), positive for KCS (item III), a positive lip biopsy (item IV, fig. 1a), positive results for the assessment of salivary glands (item V, fig. 1b, c), and positive anti-Ro/La antibodies in the sera (item VI). Primary SS is usually subclassified as glandular type and extraglandular type, and secondary SS is diagnosed when the patients fulfill the diagnostic criteria of other connective tissue diseases.

Pathomechanisms of Sjögren's Syndrome

Prevalence of SS among autoimmune diseases has been reported in the literature. One study demonstrated that more than 2 million SS patients are present in the United States [9]. Pathomechanisms of SS have also been reported in the literature. Figure 2 summarizes the current understanding of mechanisms of induction of autoimmune sialadenitis including sweat duct involvement. Most of the infiltrating cells are CD4+, CD45RO+ T cells [10]. These cells express oligoclonal T-cell receptor $V\beta_{2/13}$, produce IL6, IFN-γ, and TGF-β, and destroy epithelial cells through the FAS/FAS-L system. CD8+ T cells, although minor populations, injure the salivary glands with perforin/granzyme [11]. Tissue-specific autoantibodies such as anti-α-fodrin antibody or antimuscarine M_3-receptor antibody are also speculated to play some roles in the induction of SS [12]. Latent viral infections such as EB, HCV, HIV, and parvovirus B19 or cytomegalovirus are speculated to induce an autoimmune response as well as other collagen diseases such as

Table 1. Revised international classification criteria for SS [7]

I.	Ocular symptoms: a positive response to at least one of the following questions:
	1. Have you had daily, persistent, troublesome dry eyes for more than 3 months?
	2. Do you have a recurrent sensation of sand or gravel in the eyes?
	3. Do you use tear substitutes more than 3 times a day?
II.	Oral symptoms: a positive response to at least one of the following questions:
	1. Have you had a daily feeling of dry mouth for more than 3 months?
	2. Have you had recurrently or persistently swollen salivary glands as an adult?
	3. Do you frequently drink liquids to aid in swallowing dry food?
III.	Ocular signs – that is, objective evidence of ocular involvement defined as a positive result for at least one of the following two tests:
	1. Schirmer's I test, performed without anesthesia (5 mm in 5 min)
	2. Rose bengal score or other ocular dye score (4 according to van Bijsterveld's scoring system)
IV.	Histopathology: in minor salivary glands (obtained through normal-appearing mucosa) focal lymphocytic sialadenitis, evaluated by an expert histopathologist, with a focus score 1, defined as a number of lymphocytic foci (which are adjacent to normal-appearing mucous acini and contain more than 50 lymphocytes) per 4 mm^2 of glandular tissue [49]
V.	Salivary gland involvement: objective evidence of salivary gland involvement defined by a positive result for at least one of the following diagnostic tests:
	1. Unstimulated whole salivary flow (1.5 ml in 15 min)
	2. Parotid sialography showing the presence of diffuse sialectasis (punctate, cavitary, or destructive pattern), without evidence of obstruction in the major ducts [50]
	3. Salivary scintigraphy showing delayed uptake, reduced concentration, and/or delayed excretion of tracer [51]
VI.	Autoantibodies: presence in the serum of the following autoantibodies:
	1. Antibodies to Ro(SSA) or La(SSB) antigens, or both

rheumatoid arthritis. Recent reports suggest microchimerism of chromosome Y might be the target of an autoimmune response in a similar manner to graft-versus-host disease. In the recent reports, a significant number of Th17 cells have been shown to infiltrate the salivary glands, but their role in induction of sialadenitis has not been fully understood [13].

Cutaneous Manifestations of Sjögren's Syndrome

We made a retrospective analysis from 1990 to 1996 on the cutaneous manifestations of the patients with SS who visited the outpatient clinic at Tokyo Medical and Dental University. Table 2 shows the prevalence of cutaneous manifestations observed in primary SS at the first consultation or during the clinical course [14]. Most frequent skin manifestations are pernio-like erythema followed by angular cheilitis with red flat tongue (fig. 3a), blepharitis (fig. 3b), dry skin with macular amyloidosis (fig. 3c), AE, and drug eruptions. In addition to these cutaneous manifestations, we reported that asteatotic eczema and cutaneous amyloidosis are possibly related to hypohidrosis or impaired sweating functions.

Among these skin manifestations, we would like to focus on the clinical characteristics of hypohidrosis or anhidrosis and related skin dryness. These skin manifestations might be useful clues for the diagnosis of SS in dermatological fields.

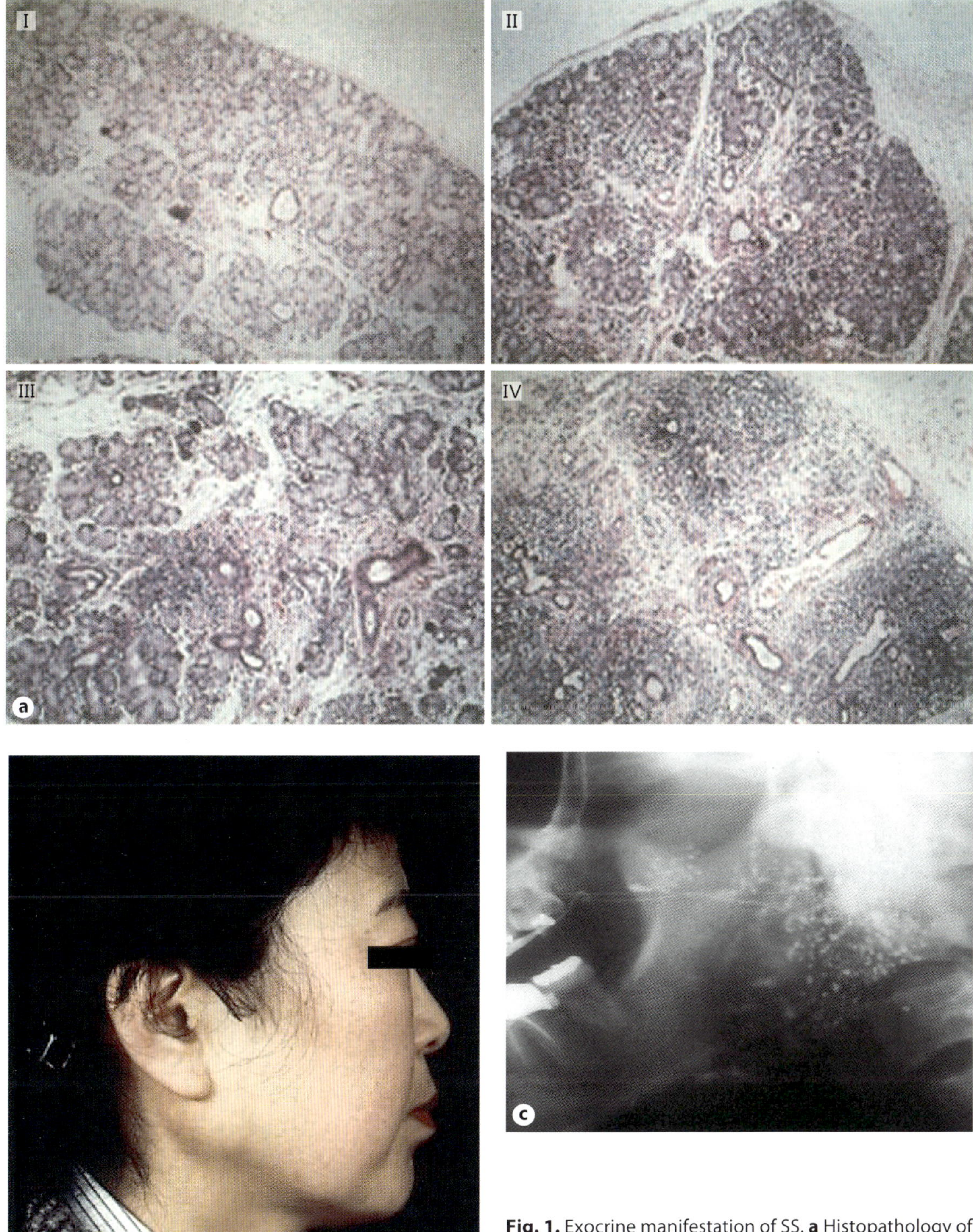

Fig. 1. Exocrine manifestation of SS. **a** Histopathology of labial salivary gland (grades I–IV). **b** Parotid gland swelling. **c** Sialography (stage 3, apple tree pattern).

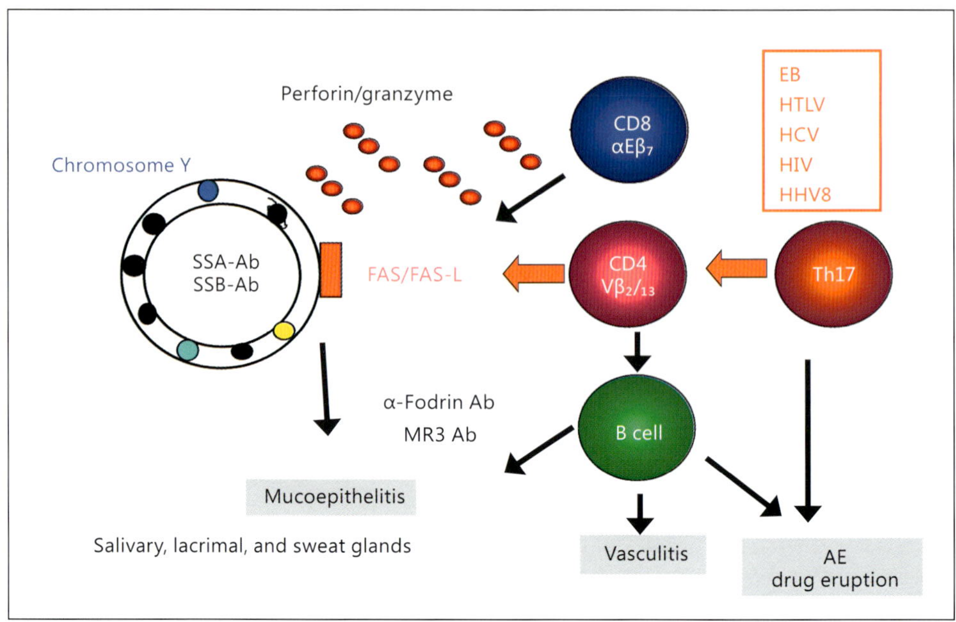

Fig. 2. Pathomechanisms of SS. Most of the infiltrating cells are CD4+, CD45RO+ T cells. These cells produce IL6, IL16, IFN-γ, and TGF-β, and destruct epithelial cells through the FAS/FAS-L system. CD8 T cells, although minor populations, injure the salivary glands with perforin/granzyme. Tissue-specific autoantibodies such as anti-α-fodrin antibody or anti-M_3 muscarine receptor antibody are also speculated to play some role in induction of SS. Latent viral infections such as EB, HCV, HIV, parvovirus B19, or cytomegalovirus are speculated to induce an autoimmune response. Recent reports suggest microchimerism of chromosome Y might be the target of autoimmune response in a similar manner to graft-versus-host disease.

Impaired Sweating as an Exocrine Manifestation in Sjögren's Syndrome

Xerophthalmia or xerostomia are important symptoms affecting the quality of life of patients with SS. CD4+ or CD8+ T cells infiltrating lacrimal or salivary glands are thought to destroy glandular cells resulting in sicca symptoms in SS. In addition to these sicca symptoms described in the diagnosis criteria, hypohidrosis and anhidrosis associated with SS have rarely been reported in the literature. These cutaneous manifestations related to sweat gland involvement in SS are not fully recognized in the field of rheumatologists and are underestimated. To examine the prevalence of hypohidrosis and to evaluate sweating as an exocrinopathy in SS, 49 patients with SS (primary form: 38; secondary form: 11) were studied [15]. Sweating was induced by mental stimulation such as deep breathing or hand grasping. Statistically significant reductions of sweat volume were seen in SS. In a control study, only hemodialysis patients showed impairment of sweating and this was greater than in patients with SS aged under 50 years (fig. 4). Patients under 50 years of age showed impaired sweat function compared with normal controls (fig. 4). Urinary β_2-microglobulin, salivary flow, and lacrimal flow showed negative correlations with sweat volume. These results suggest that patients with SS develop impaired sweating as an exocrine manifestation in addition to the known symptoms of xerostomia and xerophthalmia. Recent studies have demon-

Table 2. Cutaneous manifestations in SS (adapted from [14])

Cutaneous manifestations	Primary SS (n = 77)	Secondary SS (n = 25)	Total (n = 102)
1 Related to glandular manifestations			
Cheilitis	17	9	26
Blepharitis	15	2	17
Xerotic eczema/dry skin	7	6	13
Prurigo (?)	3	4	7
Ranula	3	0	3
2 Related to B lymphocyte activation			
Pernio-like erythema	19	7	26
Raynaud phenomenon	2	14	16
Livedo	3	3	6
Stasis dermatitis	4	1	5
Vasculitis/skin Ulcer	2	3	5
Purpura	2	1	3
Mucinosis	2	0	2
Drug eruption	8	2	10
Cutaneous amyloidosis	4	2	6
Mosquito allergy	2	0	2
Lymphoma	1	1	2
Exudative erythema (?)	5	4	9
Erythema nodosum	1	0	1
3 Related to aberrant immune response			
Alopecia	7	4	11
Lichen planus	6	1	7
Psoriasis	4	1	5
Vitiligo	2	0	2
Sweet disease	1	0	1
Sarcoidosis	0	0	0
Contact dermatitis	4	1	5
4 Infection			
Herpes infection	5	0	5
Erysipelas	2	0	2
Tuberculid	1	0	1
5 Other			
Melanosis (facial pigmentation)	4	4	8
AE	8	0	8
Tongue cancer	1	0	1

strated that water-specific channel proteins play important roles in water trafficking in the lacrimal and salivary glands in SS. These channel proteins are designated as aquaporin (AQP) and 13 AQP members are known at present. Among these AQPs, AQP5 labelling of the salivary glands from SS patients is higher at the basement membrane and lower at the apical membrane of acinar cells, which contrasts to normal distribution patterns of the glands from normal subjects [16].

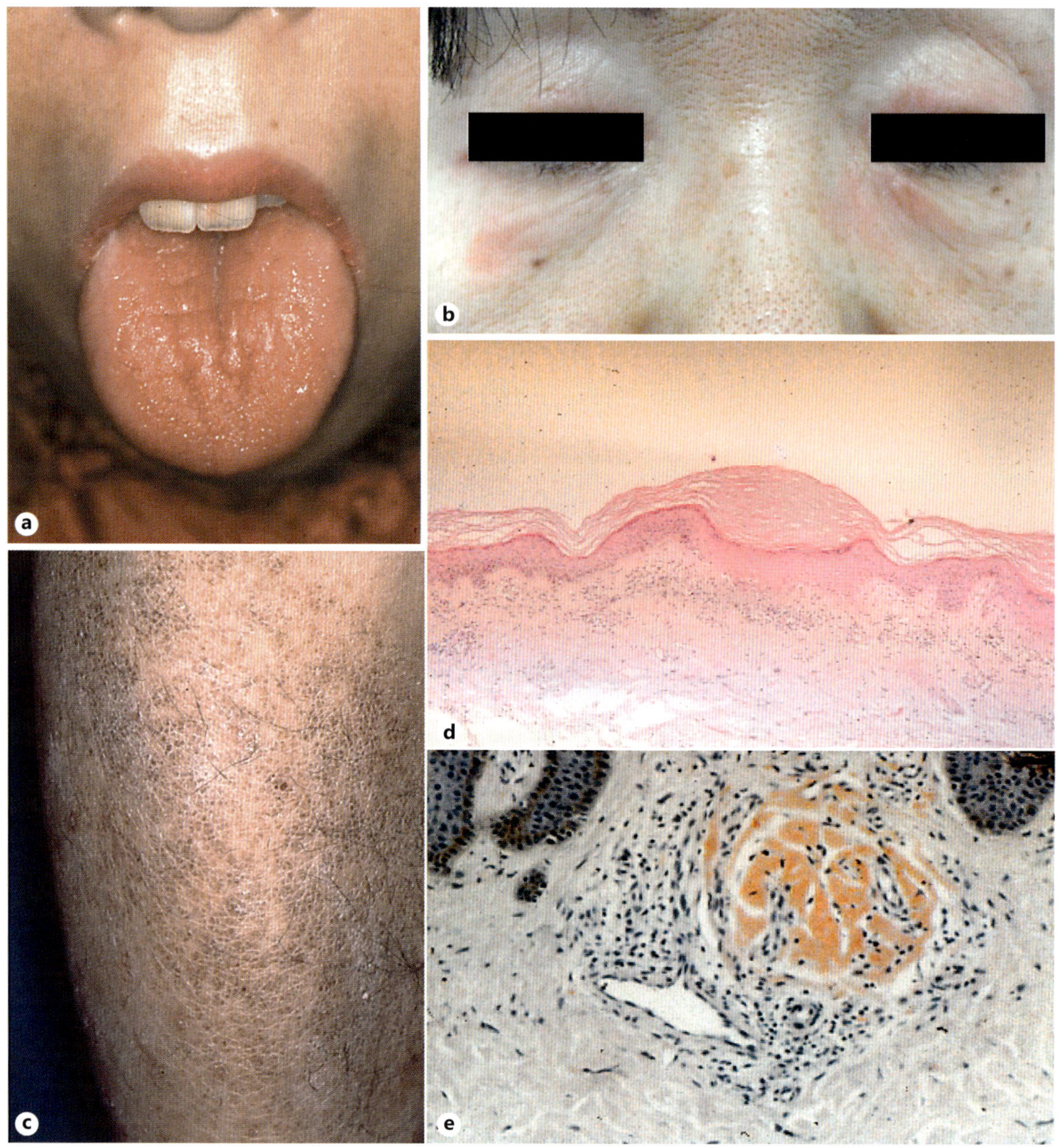

Fig. 3. Glandular manifestations of SS: bleparitis (**a**), red flat tongue and lip-stick-on-the-tooth sign (**b**), and macular amyloidosis (**c**). Clinical manifestation of **c** with pigmented macular lesions: histopathology H&E stain ×40 (**d**) and Dylon stain ×100 (**e**).

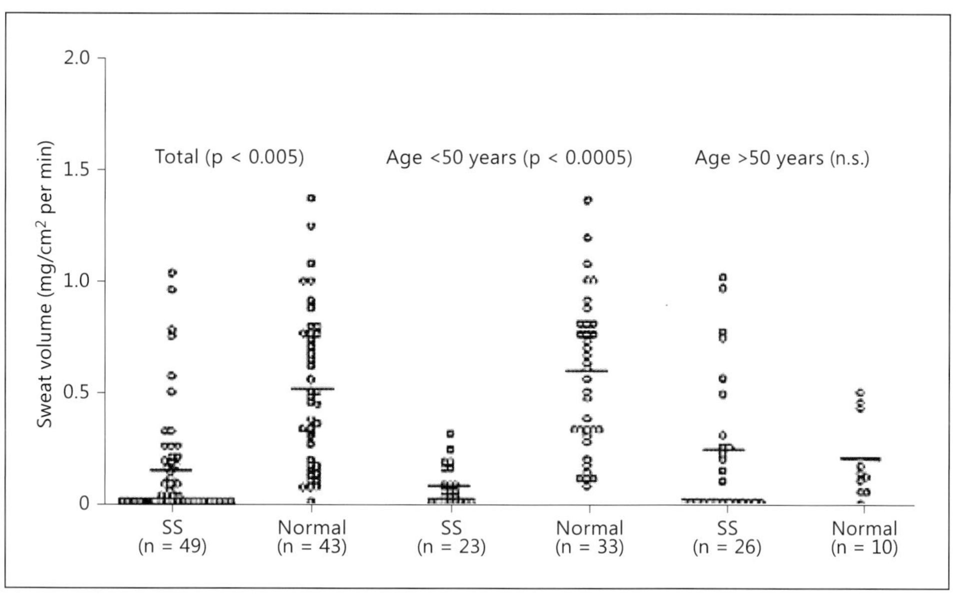

Fig. 4. Psychogenic stimulation-induced sweating in SS. Statistically significant reductions of sweat volume were seen in SS ($p < 0.005$). Patients under 50 years of age showed impaired sweat function compared with normal controls ($p < 0.0005$) [15].

This aberrant distribution pattern of AQP5 might be responsible for sicca symptoms seen in SS; however, distribution of AQP5 in sweat glands has not been reported to date.

In addition to the psychogenic sweating, we performed acetylcholine-induced sweating function in SS. Briefly, the subjects were asked to remain quiet for 60 min before undergoing the Quantitative Sudomotor Axon Reflex Test (QSART) in a climatic chamber (24 ± 0.5 °C chamber temperature and 40 ± 0.3% relative humidity, with air velocity of <1 m s^{-1}). The multicompartmental sweat capsule used in QSART consists of three concentric compartments, as shown in figure 5. Acetylcholine (100 mg ml^{-1}) iontophoretically applied to the skin from the outer compartment stimulates the underlying sweat glands directly (DIR sweating), while the glands of the skin in the central compartment of the capsule are activated indirectly via axon reflex (AXR sweating). A middle compartment separates the outer and central compartment to avoid diffusion of acetylcholine. The central compartment of the capsule serves as the site for AXR sweat volume measurement during 5 min of iontophoresis. Data for DIR sweating were obtained over the subsequent 5 min. Sweating rates were measured by the capacitance hygrometer ventilated capsule method [17]. In brief, nitrogen gas was introduced into each compartment at a constant flow rate of 0.3 liters min^{-1}, and the change in the relative humidity of effluent gas was detected by a hygrometer (model H211; Technol Seven, Yokohama, Japan). Sweat onset time, i.e. the latency period for sweating after current loading (latency time), and sweat volume over 5 min were measured, and the area under the sweating curve was calculated during 0–5 min for AXR sweating and 6–11 min for DIR sweating. Sweat production was measured on the volar forearms in the SS and control groups. Similar results were obtained in a similar manner to decreased sweat-

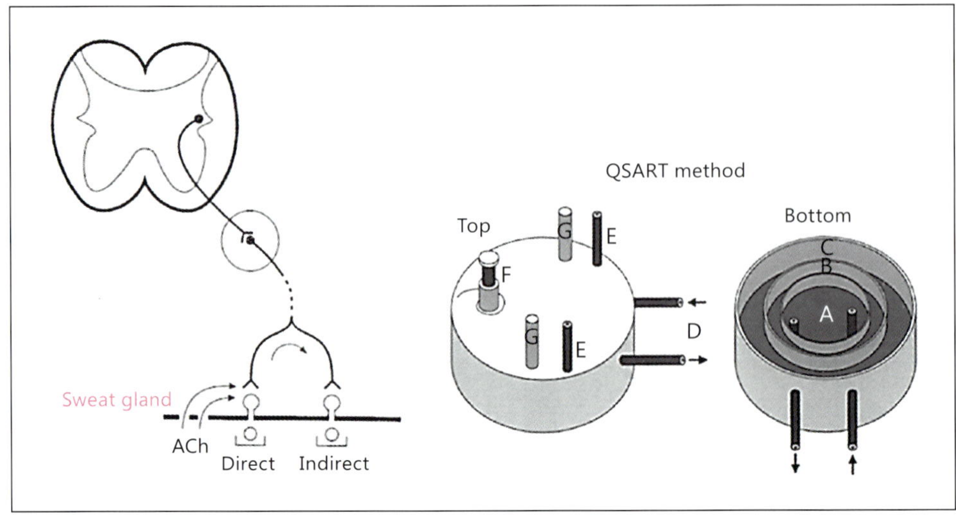

Fig. 5. AXR-mediated sweating and QSART. The DIR response is recorded from compartment C which contains acetylcholine (ACh) solution during stimulation. The AXR is recorded from A, and DIR from C after substituting a dry capsule and drying the skin [17, 46, 47].

ing functions measured by the QSART method. In SS, direct sweating as well as AXR-mediated sweating were impaired, which suggests that autoimmune mechanisms might induce impaired sweating in SS, which requires systemic steroid therapy [18].

Sweating Functions in Sjögren's Syndrome Complicated with Atopic Dermatitis

Although the prevalence of adult atopic dermatitis (AD) in Japan is 6.9% [48], complication of AD by SS is relatively rare and few case reports are available in the literature except in the setting of systemic lupus erythematosus [19, 20]. The involvement of Th17 cells in both SS [21] and AD [22] as well as the Th1 and Th2 balance theory are thought to be responsible for the rare complication of these allergic and systemic autoimmune diseases.

In SS, sweating induced by both the direct action of acetylcholine and AXR is impaired, possibly due to eccrine gland dysfunction resulting from autoimmune mechanisms mediated by CD8 T cells [23] or M_3-receptor-specific autoantibodies [24] as previously described. In contrast to SS, the reduced sweating function seen in AD is restricted only to AXR-induced indirect sweating, which is usually restored to normal levels after improvement of the dermatitis [17]. Therefore, the xerotic skin lesions seen in the present cases might be due to additive AD- and SS-related hypohidrosis with accelerated dry skin. It is well known that dry skin is occasionally seen in SS and clinical use of muscarinic M_3-receptor agonists occasionally improves this condition through recovery of sweating function [25]. In regard to the sweating function in AD, it is well known that sweating may cause itching and secondary eczema; however, the results of previous studies on sweat gland function in AD are controversial. Sweat secretion has been reported to be decreased [26, 27], increased [28, 29], and normal [30] in various experimental studies of AD. Our previous observation on sweating function using QSART clearly demonstrated that reversible impairment of sweating function is present in AD.

Most previous investigations assessed sweating function using a direct stimulation sweating test in which an intradermal acetylcholine injection resulted in direct sweat responses [25–27]. To clarify sweat function in AD, we evaluated the postganglionic sweat output, which reflects AXR-mediated sweating function, using QSART [31]. In the present cases, AXR sweat volumes were reduced and the latency time was prolonged in both nonlesional and lesional skin of AD/SS patients compared to those in nonatopic controls, and the reduction was greater in AD/SS (fig. 6). In contrast to patients with AD, the DIR response characterized by exocrine gland dysfunction in patients with SS [15, 32, 33] was significantly reduced compared to that in normal AD skin or healthy controls. The reason for normal DIR in normal skin of AD/SS patients is unclear at present. The presence of atopic skin lesions may modulate sweating function in normal skin of AD/SS patients by possible compensatory mechanisms. Recent reports have suggested that the barrier function recovers, including transepidermal water loss, or that ceramide content in the stratum corneum returns to normal levels when eczematous changes resolve [34, 35]. Possible tolerance to cholinergic stimulation, manifesting as a higher sudomotor nerve excitation threshold or negative feedback, may be controlled in patients with severe AD by psychosomatic or unknown factors that could be therapeutic targets in adults with refractory disease. Although complication of AD by SS disease has been rarely documented, it might be underestimated or overlooked in daily practice. For skin care in AD, the complication of SS should be monitored, especially in adult AD patients.

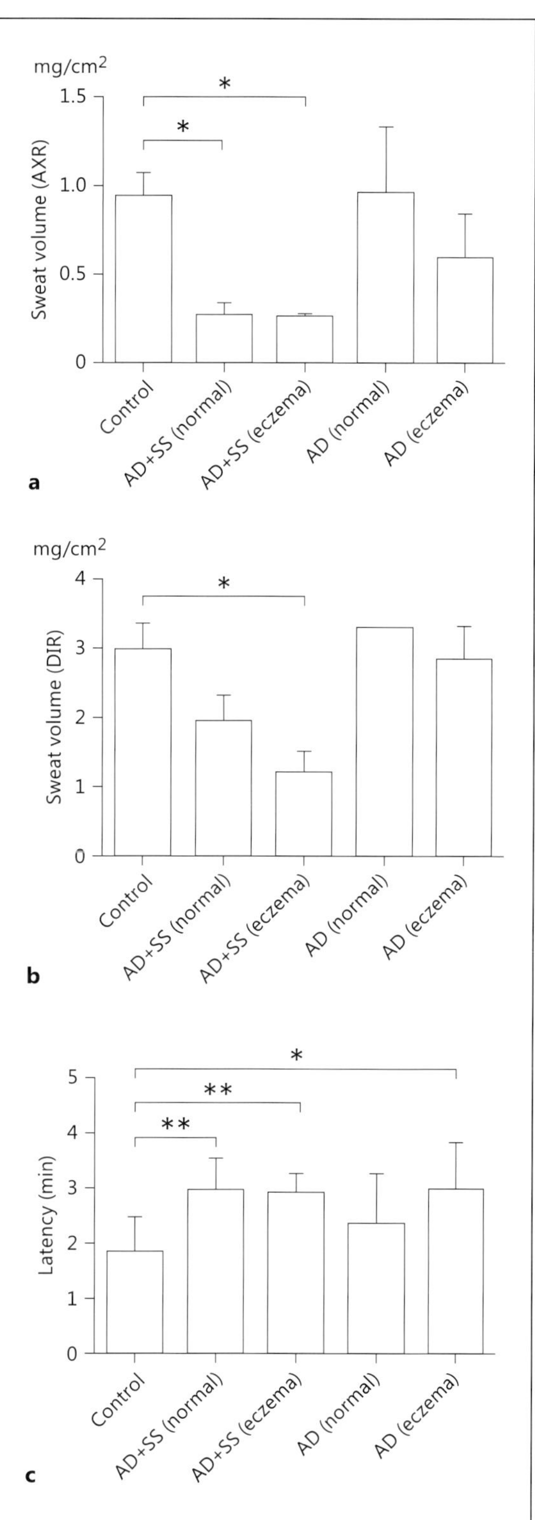

Fig. 6. Sweating functions in SS/AD overlap syndrome (unpublished observations). **a** AXR-mediated sweating. **b** Direct sweating by iontophoretically applied acetylcholine. **c** Latent time before sweating. * $p < 0.05$; ** $p < 0.01$.

Prevalence of Eyelid Dermatitis in Primary Sjögren's Syndrome

SS is an autoimmune disease characterized by CD4+ T-cell infiltration to exocrine organs such as lacrimal, salivary, or other organs, resulting in exocrine manifestations clinically including cutaneous manifestations [36–38]. Oral or ocular dryness are frequent complaints of SS patients in addition to hypohidrosis. Angular cheilitis and red flat tongue with positive 'lip-stick-on-the-tooth sign' (fig. 3a) [39] are well-known dermatological manifestations of sicca symptoms. We reported that eyelid dermatitis is another important manifestation of sicca symptoms which had not been recognized previously [40]. Fifty-two patients with primary definite SS (4 men, 48 women; mean age 54 years) were enrolled in the study, and the prevalence of eyelid dermatitis was investigated. A patch test was performed using ICDRG-European standard allergens and/or eye drops, hair dye, and cosmetics. Of the 52 patients, 22 showed eyelid dermatitis. These changes were much more frequent in elderly patients and showed a good correlation with the presence of ocular dry sensation. No significant difference was observed in clinical and other laboratory findings between patients with or without eyelid dermatitis. Although 8 of the 13 patients showed a positive patch test reaction to various allergens, no close relationship existed between the use of a suspected substance and the onset or severity of eyelid dermatitis. These results suggest that the presence of rubbing dermatitis of the eyelid may be one of the cutaneous manifestations of SS. The eyelid dermatitis seen in SS and AD especially treated with topical steroids in addition to elderly patients is a relatively heterogenous and troublesome disease. Most cases seem to be diagnosed as idiopathic blepharitis, except atopic blepharitis, and show resistance to standard dermatologic therapy. Use of eye drops and nonsteroidal emollient prevent intractable eyelid dermatitis and red face syndrome [41].

Future Perspectives

Sweat secretion from eccrine glands is controlled by the sudomotor fibers of the sympathetic nervous system through postganglionic fiber stimulation of sweat glands by acetylcholine, which reflects autonomic nervous system function. Low et al. [42] reported that when postganglionic sudomotor fibers are damaged, the AXR sweat response occurs earlier than the DIR response. Therefore, evaluating the AXR response appears to be more reliable than evaluating the DIR response. Several reports concluded that the impaired sweating observed in AD is induced by damage to eccrine glands and/or ductal components secondary to dermal or epidermal inflammation [43, 44]. The results of nearly normal DIR responses in AD patients in the present study may contradict this inflammation theory because AD patients showed nearly normal sweating in response to direct acetylcholine stimulation, which excludes the occurrence of obstruction of the sweat ducts or hypoproduction of sweat by eccrine glands. In contrast to patients with AD, the DIR response in patients with SS, which is characterized by exocrine gland dysfunction [15, 32, 33], was significantly reduced when compared with the response in healthy controls. The lack of obstruction of the sweat ducts in serial sections of lesional AD skin would also exclude the presence of organic changes in eccrine sweat ducts, although electron microscopic examination was not performed in this study. We conclude that the sweat glands are functionally intact in AD while the autonomic nervous system is disturbed in lesional and nonlesional AD skin. Possible tolerance to cholinergic stimulation, manifesting as a higher sudomotor nerve excitation threshold or negative feedback, may be controlled in patients with severe AD by psychosomatic or unknown factors that could be therapeutic targets in adults with refractory disease. Further studies are needed to elucidate autonomic nervous system function in this regard. Finally, in clinical practice, sweating is cited as the major exacerbating factor in adults with refractory AD. This contradictory result might be explained by the compensation theory of sweating. Shih et al. [45] reported that individuals who experience hyperhidrosis of the palms and soles had a much smaller sweating response on the forehead, upper chest, and arms. It is possible that total sweating volumes from the skin surface in humans are equal, i.e. if sweating from one part of the skin decreases, then sweating elsewhere increases in compensation. We only measured sweating on the volar aspect of the forearm in this investigation. Therefore, increased sweating might have been observed if sweating were recorded on the flexor aspect of the elbow or neck, where eczematous lesions commonly appear in AD. This possibility should be clarified in the future for a better understanding of the pathogenesis and treatment of refractory AD and SS.

References

1 Katayama I, Teramoto N, Arai H, et al: Annular erythema: a comparative study of Sjögren's syndrome with subacute cutaneous lupus erythematosus. Int J Dermatol 1991;30:635–639.
2 Katayama I, Yamamoto T, Otoyama K, Matsunaga T, Nishioka K: Clinical and immunological analysis of annular erythema associated with Sjögren's syndrome. Dermatology 1994;189(suppl 1):14–17.
3 Ostlere LS, Harris D, Rustin MH: Urticated annular erythema: a new manifestation of Sjogren's syndrome. Clin Exp Dermatol 1993;18:50–51.
4 Haimowitz JE, McCauliffe DP, Seykora J, et al: Annular erythema of Sjögren's syndrome in a white woman. J Am Acad Dermatol 2000;42:1069–1073.
5 Ruzicka T, Faes J, Bergner T, et al: Annular erythema associated with Sjögren's syndrome: a variant of systemic lupus erythematosus. J Am Acad Dermatol 1991;25:557–560.
6 Vitali C, Moutsopoulos HM, Bombardieri S, et al: The European Community Study Group on diagnostic criteria for Sjögren's syndrome. Sensitivity and specificity of tests for ocular and oral involvement in Sjögren's syndrome. Ann Rheum Dis 1994;53:637–647.
7 Vitali C, Bombardieri S, Jonsson R, Moutsopoulos HM, et al: Classification criteria for Sjögren syndrome: a revised version of the European criteria proposed by the American-European Consensus Group. Ann Rheum Dis 2002;61: 554–558.
8 Fujibayashi K; Japanese Medical Society for Sjögren's Syndrome: Revised Japanese Criteria for Sjögren's Syndrome. Annual Report of Japanese Ministry of Health and Welfare. Tokyo, Ministry of Health and Welfare, 1999, pp 135–138.
9 Whitacre CC: Sex differences in autoimmune disease. Nat Immunol 2001;2: 777–780.
10 Polihronis M, Tapinos NI, Theocharis SE, et al: Modes of epithelial cell death and repair in Sjögren syndrome (SS). Clin Exp Immunol 1998;114:485–490.
11 Arakaki R, Ishimaru N, Saito I, et al: Development of autoimmune exocrinopathy resembling Sjögren's syndrome in adoptively transferred mice with autoreactive CD4+ T cells. Arthritis Rheum 2003;48:3603–3609.
12 Shiari R, Kobayashi I, Toita N, et al: Epitope mapping of anti-alpha-fodrin autoantibody in juvenile Sjögren's syndrome: difference in major epitopes between primary and secondary cases. J Rheumatol 2006;33:1395–1400.
13 Itoi S, Tanemura A, Ktayama I, et al: Immunohistochemical analysis of interleukin-17 producing T helper cells and regulatory T cells infiltration in annular erythema associated with Sjögren's syndrome. Ann Dermatol 2014;26:203–208.
14 Katayama I: Clinical reviews of Sjögren's syndrome: pathogenesis and management. Jpn J Dermatol 2004;114:1639–1616.
15 Katayama I, Yokozeki H, Nishioka K: Impaired sweating as an exocrine manifestation in Sjögren's syndrome. Br J Dermatol 1995;133:716–720.
16 Delporte C, Steinfeld S: Distribution and roles of aquaporins in salivary glands. Biochim Biophys Acta 2006;1758:1061–1070.
17 Eishi K, Lee JB, Bae SJ, Takenaka M, Katayama I: Impaired sweating function in adult atopic dermatitis: results of the quantitative sudomotor axon reflex test. Br J Dermatol 2002;147:683–688.
18 Maeda A, Yamanouchi H, Lee JB, Katayama I: Oral prednisolone improved acetylcholine-induced sweating in Sjögren's syndrome related anhidrosis. Clin Rheumatol 2000;19:396–397.
19 Higashi N, Kawana S: Atopic eczema complicated by systemic lupus erythematosus. Eur J Dermatol 2005;15:500–502.
20 Sekigawa I, Yoshiike T, Iida N, Hashimoto H, Ogawa H: Two cases of atopic dermatitis associated with autoimmune abnormalities. Rheumatology (Oxford) 2003;42:184–185.
21 Katsifis GE, Rekka S, Moutsopoulos NM, Pillemer S, Wahl SM: Systemic and local interleukin-17 and linked cytokines associated with Sjögren's syndrome immunopathogenesis. Am J Pathol 2009;175:1167–1177.
22 Oyoshi MK, Murphy GF, Geha RS: Filaggrin-deficient mice exhibit TH17-dominated skin inflammation and permissiveness to epicutaneous sensitization with protein antigen. J Allergy Clin Immunol 2009;124:485–493, 493.e1.
23 Katayama I, Asai T, Nishioka K, Nishiyama S: Annular erythema associated with primary Sjogren syndrome: analysis of T cell subsets in cutaneous infiltrates. J Am Acad Dermatol 1989;21: 1218–1221.

24 Naito Y, Matsumoto I, Wakamatsu E, et al: Muscarinic acetylcholine receptor autoantibodies in patients with Sjögren's syndrome. Ann Rheum Dis 2005;64: 510–511.
25 Wienrich M, Meier D, Ensinger HA, et al: Pharmacodynamic profile of the M1 agonist talsaclidine in animals and man. Life Sci 2001;68:2593–2600.
26 Parkkinen MU, Kiistala R, Kiistala U: Sweating response to moderate thermal stress in atopic dermatitis. Br J Dermatol 1992;126:346–350.
27 Greene RM, Winkelmann RK, Opfer-Gehrking TL, Low PA: Sweating patterns in atopic dermatitis patients. Arch Dermatol Res 1989;281:373–376.
28 Rovensky J, Saxl O: Differences in the dynamics of sweat secretion in atopic children. J Invest Dermatol 1964;43: 171–176.
29 Warndorff JA: The response of the sweat gland to acetylcholine in atopic subjects. Br J Dermatol 1970;83:306–311.
30 Lobitz WC Jr, Campbell CJ: Physiologic studies in atopic dermatitis (disseminated neurodermatitis). I. The local cutaneous response to intradermally injected acetyl- choline and epinephrine. AMA Arch Derm Syphilol 1953;67:575–589.
31 Kitaba S, Matsui S, Iimuro E, et al: Four cases of atopic dermatitis complicated by Sjögren's syndrome: link between dry skin and autoimmune anhidrosis. Allergol Int 2011;60:387–391.
32 Sais G, Admella C, Fantova MJ, Montero JC: Lymphocytic autoimmune hidradenitis, cutaneous leucocytoclastic vasculitis and primary Sjögren's syndrome. Br J Dermatol 1998;139:1073–1076.
33 Mitchell J, Greenspan J, Daniels T, Whitcher JP, Maibach HI: Anhidrosis (hypohidrosis) in Sjogren's syndrome. J Am Acad Dermatol 1987;16:233–235.
34 Löffler H, Effendy I: Skin susceptibility of atopic individuals. Contact Dermatitis 1999;40:239–242.
35 Matsumoto M, Sugiura H, Uehara M: Skin barrier function in patients with completely healed atopic dermatitis. J Dermatol Sci 2000;23:178–182.
36 Teramoto N, Katayama I, Arai H, et al: Annular erythema: possible association with primary Sjögren's syndrome. J Am Acad Dermatol 1989;20:596–601.
37 Katayama I: Clinical analysis of recurrent hypergammaglobulinemic purpura associated with Sjögren syndrome. J Dermatol 1995;22:186–190.
38 Katayama I, Kotobuki Y, Kiyohara E, Murota H: Annular erythema associated with Sjögren's syndrome: review of the literature on the management and clinical analysis of skin lesions. Mod Rheumatol 2010;20:123–129.
39 Ruiz-Arguelles GJ: The 'lipstick-on-teeth' sign in Sjögren's syndrome. N Engl J Med 1986;315:1030–1031.
40 Katayama I, Koyano T, Nishioka K: Prevalence of eyelid dermatitis in primary Sjögren's syndrome. Int J Dermatol 1994;33:421–424.
41 Rapaport MJ, Rapaport V: Eyelid dermatitis to red face syndrome to cure: clinical experience in 100 cases. J Am Acad Dermatol 1999;41:435–442.
42 Low PA, Zimmerman BR, Dyck PJ: Comparison of distal sympathetic with vagal function in diabetic neuropathy. Muscle Nerve 1986;9:592–596.
43 Sulzberger MB, Herrmann F: Clinical significance of disturbances in the delivery of sweat; in Bear RL (ed): Atopic Dermatitis. New York, New York University Press, 1955, p 34.
44 Papa CM, Kligman AM: Mechanism of eccrine anhidrosis. I. High level blockade. J Invest Dermatol 1966;47:1–9.
45 Shih CJ, Wu JJ, Lin MT: Autonomic dysfunction in palmar hyperhidrosis. J Auton Nerv Syst 1983;8:33–34.
46 Kihara M, Opfer-Gehrking TL, Low PA: Comparison of directly stimulated with axon-reflex-mediated sudomotor responses in human subjects and in patients with diabetes. Muscle Nerve 1993; 16: 655–660.
47 Lee J-B, Matsumoto T, Othman T et al: Suppression of the sweat gland sensitivity to acetylcholine applied iontophoretically in tropical Africans compared to temperate Japanese. Trop Med 1997;39:111–121.
48 Saeki H, Tsunemi Y, Fujita H, et al: Prevalence of atopic dermatitis determined by clinical examination in Japanese adults. J Dermatol 2006;33:817–819.
49 Daniels TE, Whitcher JP: Association of patterns of labial salivary gland inflammation with keratoconjunctivitis sicca. Analysis of 618 patients with suspected Sjögren's syndrome. Arthritis Rheum 1994;37:869–877.
50 Rubin H, Holt M: Secretory sialography in diseases of the major salivary glands. AJR Am J Roentgenol 1957;77:575–98.
51 Shall GL, Anderson LG, Wolf RO, Herdt JR, Tarpley TM Jr, Cummings NA, et al: Xerostomia in Sjögren's syndrome: evaluation by sequential scintigraphy. JAMA 1971;216:2109–2116.

Ichiro Katayama
Department of Dermatology
Course of Integrated Medicine
Graduate School of Medicine
Osaka University
2-2 Yamadaoka, Suita-shi
Osaka 565-0871 (Japan)
E-Mail katayama@derma.med.osaka-u.ac.jp

Yokozeki H, Murota H, Katayama I (eds): Perspiration Research.
Curr Probl Dermatol. Basel, Karger, 2016, vol 51, pp 75–79 (DOI: 10.1159/000446781)

Clinical Analysis and Management of Acquired Idiopathic Generalized Anhidrosis

Takahiro Satoh

Department of Dermatology, National Defense Medical College, Tokorozawa, Japan

Abstract

Acquired idiopathic generalized anhidrosis (AIGA) is a sweating disorder characterized by inadequate sweating in response to heat stimuli such as high temperature, humidity, and physical exercise. Patients exhibit widespread nonsegmental hypohidrosis/anhidrosis without any apparent cause, but the palms, soles, and axillae are rarely affected. Heat stroke readily develops due to increased body temperature. AIGA commonly affects young males. Approximately 30–60% of patients show complications of cholinergic urticaria, also known as idiopathic pure sudomotor failure or hypohidrotic cholinergic urticaria. Systemic corticosteroids are the most effective therapy, although recurrence is not uncommon.

Acquired idiopathic generalized anhidrosis (AIGA) is a rare disorder characterized by an inability to sweat in the absence of apparent causative skin, metabolic, or neurological etiologies. This disorder typically affects young males and severely disturbs quality of life. When exposed to circumstances of high temperature, patients with AIGA easily succumb to heat stroke, displaying symptoms such as general malaise, hyperthermia, dizziness, palpitations, faintness, and ultimately loss of consciousness due to dysregulation of body temperature.

Epidemiology

The actual incidence of the disease is unknown. According to an epidemiological study conducted in 2011 [1] by a Japanese study group supported by the Ministry of Health, Labour and Welfare in Japan, 145 patients were diagnosed with AIGA in 94 university medical institutes in Japan during the preceding 5 years. Mean age was 30.3 years (range: 1–69), with incidence peaking at 10–30 years of age. A significant male predominance was evident (126 males, 19 females). Another study in a single institute also reported a significant male predominance with a mean age of 33.1 years [2]. The majority of AIGA patients reported previously have shown preferential, but not exclusive, Asian ethnicity, and incidences and clinical characteristics in the United States and European countries thus remain uncertain.

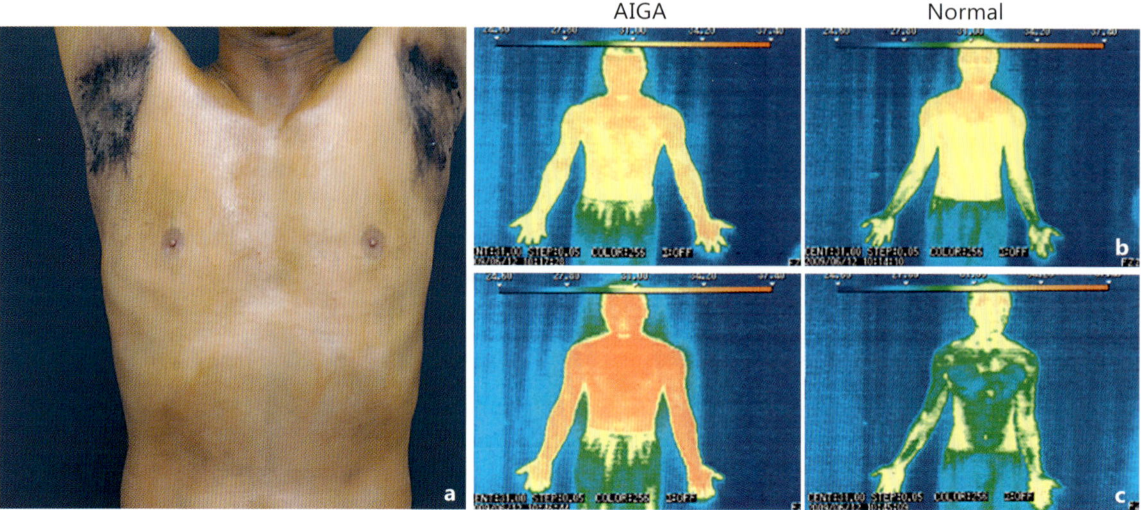

Fig. 1. Results of the starch-iodine test (left) and thermography (right). **a** Sweating in an AIGA patient was only detected at the axillae and anterior neck. Unlike a healthy control (normal), the patient (AIGA) showed increased body temperature after exercise. **b** Before exercise. **c** After exercise.

Clinical Manifestations and Diagnosis

Patients with AIGA are unable to show adequate sweating in response to heat stimuli such as high temperature, humidity, and physical exercise. Anhidrosis/hypohidrosis usually occurs on the trunk in a symmetrical distribution. The extremities and occasionally the face may also be affected, but involvement of the palms, soles, or axillae is rare. Approximately 30–60% of AIGA patients complain of a tingling sensation and/or wheals under circumstances that would normally promote sweating. In 2004, Nakazato et al. [3] proposed the term 'idiopathic pure sudomotor failure (IPSF)' for the subgroup of AIGA characterized by acute or sudden onset, sharp pain or cholinergic urticaria, lack of autonomic dysfunctions other than hypohidrosis, elevated levels of immunoglobulin E, preservation of emotional sweating, and favorable response to systemic corticosteroids. IPSF represents either the same entity or a subtype of hypohidrotic cholinergic urticaria, a diagnostic term commonly used by dermatologists. Details of the relationship between IPSF and hypohidrotic cholinergic urticaria are discussed in the chapter by Tokura [this vol., pp. 94–100].

To reach a diagnosis of AIGA, congenital diseases such as hypohidrotic/anhidrotic ectodermal dysplasia, congenital insensitivity to pain with anhidrosis, and Fabry disease should be excluded. Secondary sweating disorders associated with neurological diseases, metabolic diseases, Sjögren's syndrome, and drug-induced sweating disturbances must also be ruled out. The Japan Intractable Disease Information Center proposed the following diagnostic criteria for AIGA: (1) acquired nonsegmental and widespread hypohidrosis/anhidrosis without apparent cause, and no detection of abnormal neurological or autonomic nerve functions other than those involving sweating, and (2) hypohidrosis/anhidrosis involving more than 25% of the total body surface area as detected by a starch-iodine test and/or thermography (fig. 1). These two criteria can be diagnosed as AIGA [http://www.mhlw.go.jp/file/06-

Seisakujouhou-10900000-Kenkoukyoku/0000085405.pdf (in Japanese)]. Although AIGA is a sweating disorder, patients are occasionally unaware of the impaired sweating, and may present with chief complaints of various symptoms of heatstroke and/or cholinergic urticaria.

Histopathology

Histopathological findings of AIGA are inconsistent. While some patients show no abnormalities, others exhibit weak or mild lymphocytic cellular infiltrates around secretory portions/ducts [2, 4, 5]. Atrophy of the eccrine apparatus may be evident. Infiltrative lymphocytes comprise CD4+ and CD8+ T cells and a mixture of CXCR3+ Th1 cells and CCR4+ Th2 cells [6]. Another report described IL-17+ cells around eccrine glands [7]. Poral occlusion by keratotic plugs may also be seen [8] (fig. 2).

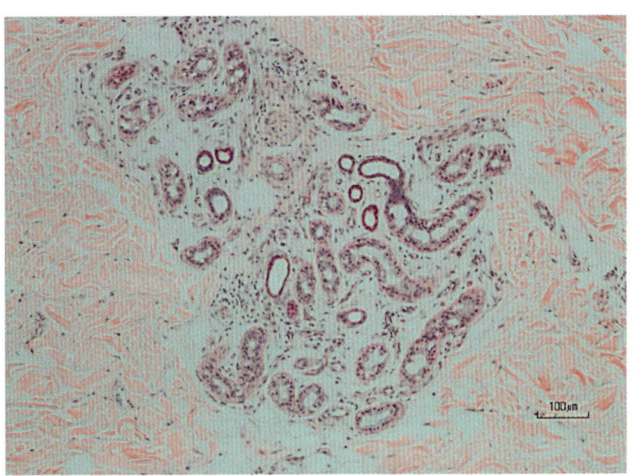

Fig. 2. Histopathological features of a patient with IPSF. Mononuclear cell infiltration is apparent around eccrine glands.

Etiology

AIGA seems to be a disease of heterogeneous etiologies. Theoretically, the following mechanisms can be considered: (1) dysfunction or degeneration of cholinergic sympathetic nerve fibers involved in sweating (sudomotor neuropathy), (2) dysfunction of acetylcholine receptors and/or cholinergic signals (IPSF could be included in this category), and (3) primary failures of the sweat glands with apparent morphological changes of the sweat apparatus. Poral occlusion mediated by hyperkeratosis of the acrosyringium has been implicated as one mechanism underlying acquired hypohidrosis with cholinergic urticaria [9], but whether hyperkeratosis of the intraepidermal sweat gland epithelium causes arrest of sweat flow and thus leads to generalized anhidrosis remains uncertain. One previous report has demonstrated autoantibodies against cholinergic receptor M_3 in 1 of 12 AIGA patients [5]. In an investigation of AIGA with cholinergic urticaria or IPSF [3], decreased expression of cholinergic receptor M_3 was found in the inner cells of sweat glands [10]. Detailed immunopathological features of hypohidrotic cholinergic urticaria are described in the chapter by Tokura [this vol., pp. 94–100].

Treatments

It is essential to advise patients to maintain careful control of their body temperature by means such as avoiding heated circumstances, usage of air-conditioning, carrying a water bottle to avoid dehydration, and cooling the neck and axillae with chilled water in portable bottles under hot and/or humid conditions.

Although no randomized controlled study has been performed to date, various case reports have demonstrated clinical effects of systemic corticosteroids, particularly in the form of intravenous pulse therapy occasionally followed by oral corticosteroids with gradually tapering dosages [2, 7, 8] (fig. 3). However, recurrence is not uncommon. One report described 2 patients with AIGA successfully treated using oral antihistamines [11]

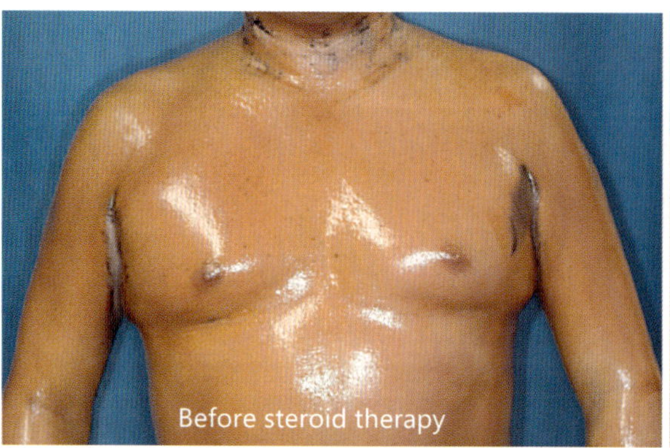

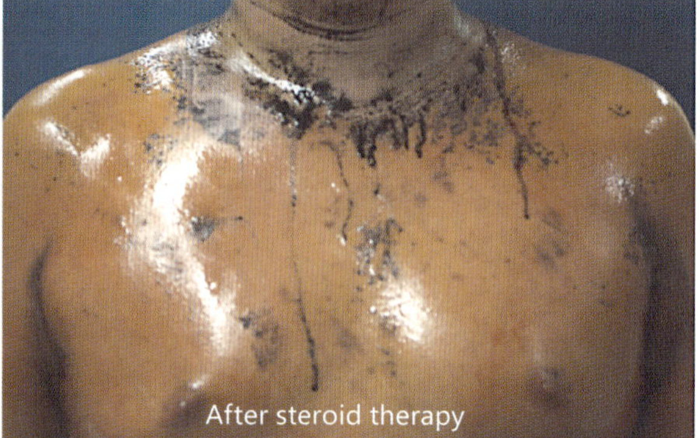

Fig. 3. Effects of steroid pulse therapy. Sweating function is improved as shown by the results of the starch-iodine test.

based on evidence that histamine inhibits the acetylcholine-induced sweating function of eccrine glands [12]. Another group recently administered intravenous immunoglobulin to treat and prevent the recurrence of AIGA [13]. Use of immunosuppressants such as cyclosporine, acetylcholine receptor agonists (e.g. pilocarpine hydrochloride and cevimeline hydrochloride hydrate), and Chinese herbal medicines has also been an option, but the clinical effects appear inconsistent.

Conclusion

Pathological etiologies of AIGA may be heterogeneous. Although systemic corticosteroids represent the most effective therapeutic option, physicians have encountered many patients with recurrence and/or extreme resistance to corticosteroids. Establishment of novel alternative therapies is imperative, as patients with AIGA experience great difficulties in daily life.

References

1 Satoh T, Yokozeki H, Asahina M, Katayama I, Nakazato Y, Watanabe D, et al: Establishment of the Guidelines for the Pathological Analysis and Treatment of Acquired Idiopathic Generalized Anhidrosis. Health, Labour Sciences Research Grant for Research on Measures for Intractable Disease General and Group Research Report in 2011. Tokyo, Ministry of Health, Labour and Welfare, 2012, pp 28–37.

2 Ohshima Y, Yanagishita T, Ito K, Tamada Y, Nishimura N, Inukai Y, et al: Treatment of patients with acquired idiopathic generalized anhidrosis. Br J Dermatol 2013;168:430–432.

3 Nakazato Y, Tamura N, Ohkuma A, Yoshimaru K, Shimazu K: Idiopathic pure sudomotor failure: anhidrosis due to deficits in cholinergic transmission. Neurology 2004;63:1476–1480.

4 Tay LK, Chong WS: Acquired idiopathic anhidrosis: a diagnosis often missed. J Am Acad Dermatol 2014;71:499–506.

5 Asahina M, Sano K, Fujinuma Y, Kuwabara S: Investigation of antimuscarinic receptor autoantibodies in patients with acquired idiopathic generalized anhidrosis. Internal Med 2013;52:2733–2737.

6 Sawada Y, Nakamura M, Bito T, Sakabe J, Kabashima-Kubo R, Hino R, et al: Decreased expression of acetylcholine esterase in cholinergic urticaria with hypohidrosis or anhidrosis. J Invest Dermatol 2014;134:276–279.

7 Iwama E, Fujimura T, Tanita K, Ishibashi M, Watabe A, Aiba S: Acquired idiopathic generalized anhidrosis: an immunohistopathological investigation of peri-glands infiltrated with immunoreactive cells. Acta Derm Venereol 2015; 95:743–744.

8 Fukunaga A, Horikawa T, Sato M, Nishigori C: Acquired idiopathic generalized anhidrosis: possible pathogenic role of mast cells. Br J Dermatol 2009; 160:1337–1340.

9 Chinuki Y, Tsumori T, Yamamoto O, Morita E: Cholinergic urticaria associated with acquired hypohidrosis: an ultrastructural study. Acta Derm Venereol 2011;91:197–198.

10 Sawada Y, Nakamura M, Bito T, Fukamachi S, Kabashima R, Sugita K, et al: Cholinergic urticaria: studies on the muscarinic cholinergic receptor M_3 in anhidrotic and hypohidrotic skin. J Invest Dermatol 2010;130:2683–2686.
11 Suma A, Murota H, Kitaba S, Yamaoka T, Kato K, Matsui S, et al: Idiopathic pure sudomotor failure responding to oral antihistamine with sweating activities. Acta Derm Venereol 2014;94:723–724.
12 Matsui S, Murota H, Takahashi A, Yang L, Lee JB, Omiya K, et al: Dynamic analysis of histamine-mediated attenuation of acetylcholine-induced sweating via GSK3beta activation. J Invest Dermatol 2014;134:326–334.
13 Masuda T, Obayashi K, Ueda M, Fujimoto A, Tasaki M, Misumi Y, et al: Therapeutic effects and prevention of recurrence of acquired idiopathic generalized anhidrosis via i.v. immunoglobulin treatment. J Dermatol 2016;43:336–337.

Takahiro Satoh, MD, PhD
Department of Dermatology
National Defense Medical College
3-2 Namiki
Tokorozawa 359-8513 (Japan)
E-Mail tasaderm@ndmc.ac.jp

Yokozeki H, Murota H, Katayama I (eds): Perspiration Research.
Curr Probl Dermatol. Basel, Karger, 2016, vol 51, pp 80–85 (DOI: 10.1159/000446785)

Dyshidrotic Eczema and Its Relationship to Metal Allergy

Aya Nishizawa

Department of Dermatology, National Defense Medical College, Tokorozawa, Japan

Abstract

Dyshidrotic eczema, also known as dyshidrotic dermatitis or pompholyx, is characterized by pruritic, small tense vesicles mainly on the palmoplantar region and lateral and ventral surfaces of the fingers. While its etiology appears to be related to sweating, as dyshidrotic eczema often occurs in an individual with hyperhidrosis, and the spring allergy season, histologic examination shows an eczematous reaction around the sweat ducts which is not associated with abnormalities of the sweat ducts. More recently, the nomenclature of 'acute and recurrent vesicular hand dermatitis' has been proposed to reflect clinical features of dyshidrotic eczema. Although the exact etiology of dyshidrotic eczema remains unknown, given the presence of metal allergy in patients with dyshidrotic eczema and the improvement of the symptoms by removing metal allergen, metal allergy is regarded as one of the important potential etiologic factors for dyshidrotic eczema.

Dyshidrotic eczema, also known as dyshidrotic dermatitis or pompholyx, is characterized by pruritic, small tense vesicles mainly on the palmoplantar region and lateral and ventral surfaces of the fingers. Superficial crusting and desquamation often replace the ruptured small vesicles of dyshidrotic eczema. The exact etiology remains unknown. Most cases are idiopathic. Factors that may predispose to the development of dyshidrotic eczema in a susceptible individual include atopy, contact allergens, contact irritants, dermatophyte infection, allergy to ingested metal (in particular nickel and cobalt), hyperhidrosis, prolonged use of protective gloves, intravenous immunoglobulin, psychological stress, and smoking. While its etiology appears to be related to sweating, as dyshidrotic eczema often occurs in an individual with hyperhidrosis, and the spring allergy season, histologic examination shows an eczematous reaction around the sweat ducts which is not associated with abnormalities of the sweat ducts. More recently, the nomenclature of 'acute and recurrent vesicular hand dermatitis' has been proposed to reflect clinical features of dyshidrotic eczema [1, 2]. Fisher [3] reported a case of an individual with vesicles mainly on hands and feet which were produced by systemic contact-type dermatitis due to metal allergy induced by exposure to an allergen through the circulatory system without external exposure to an allergen. Therefore, dyshidrotic eczema can be considered to be a type of metal allergy.

In this chapter, clinical features of dyshidrotic eczema and its relationship to metal allergy are described. Also, the results of 3-dimensional analysis by optical coherence tomography (OCT) of the lesion along with histopathological analysis of the sweat ducts are shown to support the theory that dyshidrotic eczema might be provoked by a metal allergen excreted from the sweat ducts after a systemically administered allergen reached the skin.

Relationship to Metal Allergy

Metal allergy may result in allergic contact dermatitis and systemic allergic (contact) dermatitis. Contact dermatitis, triggered by external exposure to an allergen such as metals in jewelry and chromate in cement and leather, is the most common form of metal allergy. Systemic contact dermatitis or systemically reactivated allergic contact dermatitis occurs when a person who is already sensitized to an allergen through skin contact is exposed to that allergen via a systemic route such as an oral, inhalational, injectable, or transmucosal route. Allergens known to induce systemic contact dermatitis include dental filling materials and foods containing metal allergens such as nickel. Dyshidrotic eczema and palmoplantar pustulosis are types of systemic allergic dermatitis. Systemic allergic dermatitis by a metal allergen is considered to be induced by allergens excreted from the sweat ducts after orally ingested metal allergens are absorbed in the gastrointestinal tract. This has been the primary rationale for the treatment with a low-nickel diet in the management of nickel eczema [4]. However, this contention is still under discussion as no significant statistical difference in treatment effects between the groups with a low-nickel diet and those with placebo has been reported.

Testing for Metal Allergy

Patch Testing with Metal Allergens

Patch testing is a standard test for the diagnosis of metal allergy in terms of cost and safety. The readings should be done at 48 h, 72 h, and 7 days after the application of the patches. Since patch-testing contactants such as metals may develop irritant reactions, the reading for metal contactants should be done after 72 h.

While the positive rate of a patch test varies in the different types of diseases and at different institutions, a high positive rate of 67% has been reported in patch testing of patients with dyshidrotic eczema [5]. The metals which exhibit a high positive rate of patch-test reaction include nickel, cobalt, and chromium.

Oral Provocation Testing

Oral provocation testing is a useful test to establish a diagnosis of metal allergy. However, there has been no previous report of oral provocation testing with gold, mercury, arsenic, platinum, or lead since these metals are harmful to the human body and are not contained in foods, whereas oral provocation testing with nickel, cobalt, and chromium, which are contained in foods, is feasible. Christensen and Möller [6] reported a case series of flare-up reactions of dyshidrotic eczema after oral challenge with nickel. There has also been a previous report of positive oral provocation testing with nickel, cobalt, and chromium in patients with dyshidrotic eczema in which 4 of 6 patients showed vesicular reactions on their hands with

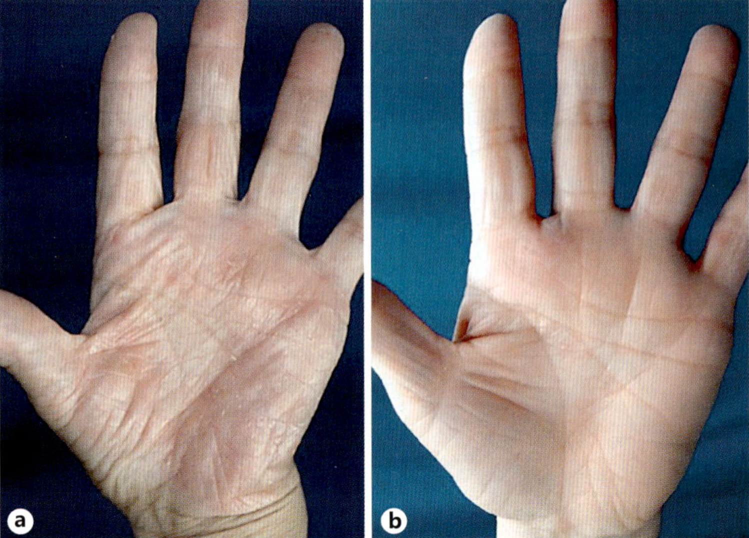

Fig. 1. A case in which skin lesions healed after dental alloys that included chromium were removed. **a** Skin lesions before treatment. **b** Skin lesions after removal of the dental alloy.

oral provocation testing with those metals [7]. Oral provocation testing with oatmeal, soybean, and chocolate containing high concentrations of metals can also be performed without oral challenge with metals. In fact, an aggravation of hand eczema and increased blood and urine nickel levels after oral challenge with a supplementary high-nickel diet has been observed in patients with vesicular hand eczema [8].

Dietary Restriction

An elimination diet can be performed to see the clinical course of eczema after removing high concentrations of specific metals from the diet, especially for patients suspected of having a metal allergy based on clinical history who cannot tolerate oral provocation testing. Oral cromoglicic acid, an antiallergic compound which reduces intestinal absorption of metals, can also be administered to see the clinical course of eczema for patients who fail to show improvement after an elimination diet.

Removal of Dental Metal

A patch test can be positive due to the presence of dental metal in the oral cavity. Therefore, it is necessary to examine the content of dental metal alloys before the interpretation of patch testing is done. In fact, the removal of the dental alloy has been reported to result in healing of the skin lesions (fig. 1). Previous reports have also shown that patients developed an eczematous reaction to the newly placed metal after the removal of the dental metal eliciting allergy. This highlights the need for assessment of dental metal used for dental filling.

Relationship to Sweat Ducts

Dyshidrotic eczema frequently affects the palmoplantar areas with the highest density of sweat ducts in the human body. Previous reports have shown a possible association between dyshidrotic eczema and sweat ducts. Also, a recent report has shown the presence of spongiotic lesions in the acrosyringium in the area of bile-colored vesicles in a patient with jaundice [9]. Nonetheless, an as-

2

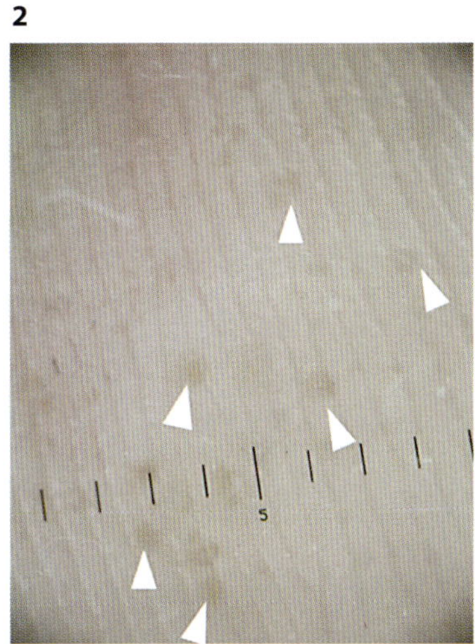

3

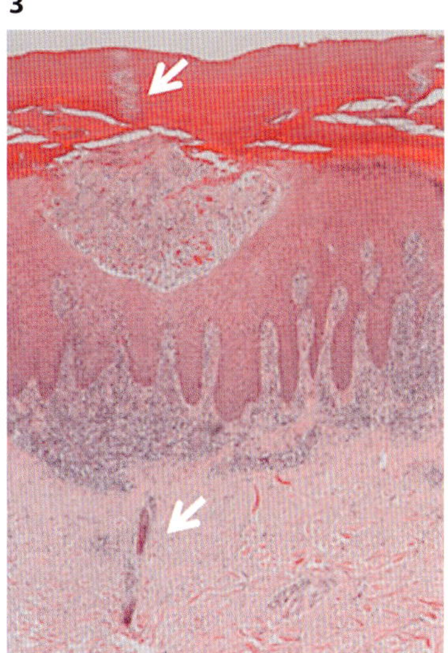

Fig. 2. Dermoscopy findings: vesicles (arrowheads) are found mainly in the crista cutis where the sweat ducts open into.

Fig. 3. Histopathological finding of the vesicles of dyshidrotic eczema: a sweat duct (arrows) passing through the vesicles is identified.

sociation between dyshidrotic eczema and sweat ducts has not been established, and the exact etiology of dyshidrotic eczema still remains unknown.

Dermoscopy Findings

An association between vesicles and sweat ducts is suggested when vesicles are seen in the crista cutis or when sweat ducts are identified in the center of vesicles. This is because sweat ducts open into the crista cutis in the palmoplantar area. In fact, vesicles are often found mainly in the crista cutis (fig. 2). Therefore, an association between vesicles and sweat ducts is often suggested.

Histopathological Findings

Histopathological analysis of the biopsy specimen from the vesicles of dyshidrotic eczema reveals the presence of sweat ducts in the stratum corneum located above the vesicles or the epidermis or dermis located underneath the vesicles (fig. 3). However, sweat ducts are also found in the area adjacent to the vesicles; moreover, often no sweat ducts are observed in the areas of vesicles.

To clarify the association between vesicles and sweat ducts, it is sometimes necessary to perform immunostains using specific antibodies against GCDFP, a specific marker for sweat ducts, and dermcidin, an antimicrobial peptide contained only in eccrine sweat glands. GCDFP immunostaining might show a spiral structure suggesting an eccrine duct in the vesicles or partial positive reaction in the vesicles. Dermcidin immunostaining might also show a similar positive reaction as seen in the GCDFP immunostain or positive reaction in the areas of vesicles (fig. 4). These findings suggest an eczematous reaction induced by sweat. Given the possible presence of metal in sweat, which induces metal allergy, these results also suggest the possible association between dyshidrotic eczema and metal allergy.

Optical Coherence Tomography

OCT is a newly developed image analyzer using optical coherence, and analyzes the dynamic changes of the lesion by obtaining 3-dimensional images of the lesion. This image analyzing system enables a researcher to investigate 3-dimensional dynamic changes of the vesicles and sweat ducts in the stratum corneum and epidermis at the

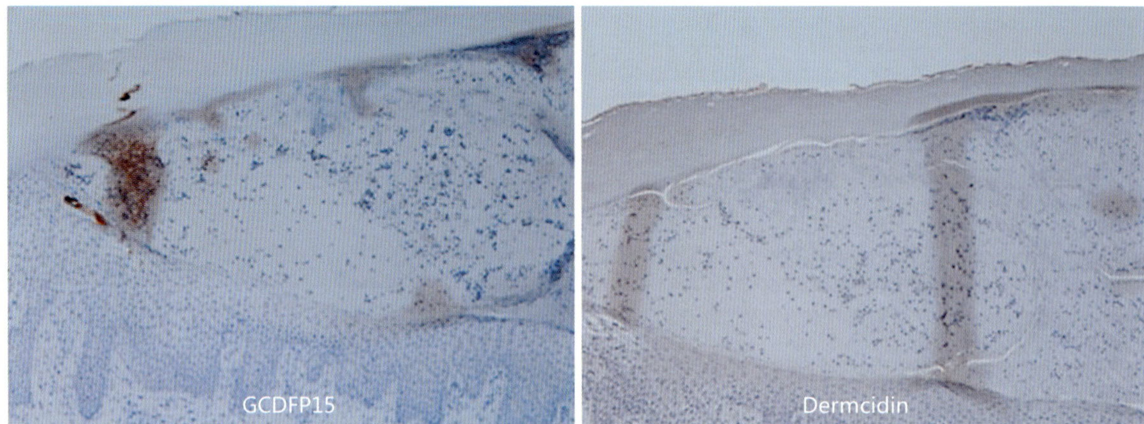

Fig. 4. GCDFP immunostaining shows a spiral structure suggesting an eccrine duct in the vesicles or partial positive reaction in the vesicles. A dermcidin immunostain also shows a similar positive reaction as seen in the GCDFP immunostain.

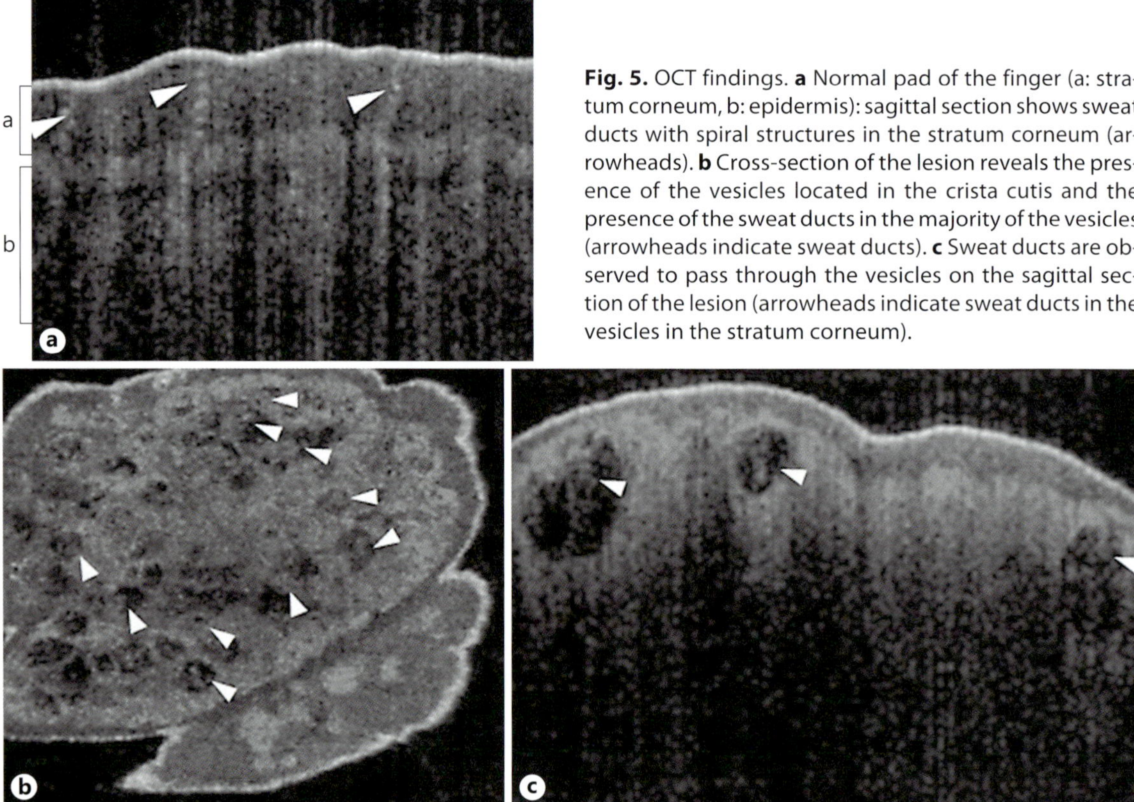

Fig. 5. OCT findings. **a** Normal pad of the finger (a: stratum corneum, b: epidermis): sagittal section shows sweat ducts with spiral structures in the stratum corneum (arrowheads). **b** Cross-section of the lesion reveals the presence of the vesicles located in the crista cutis and the presence of the sweat ducts in the majority of the vesicles (arrowheads indicate sweat ducts). **c** Sweat ducts are observed to pass through the vesicles on the sagittal section of the lesion (arrowheads indicate sweat ducts in the vesicles in the stratum corneum).

same time. OCT of the cross-section of the lesion in dyshidrotic eczema reveals the presence of the vesicles located in the crista cutis and the presence of sweat ducts in the majority of the vesicles. Moreover, sweat ducts have been observed to pass through the vesicles on the sagittal section of the lesion (fig. 5). OCT can analyze 3-dimensional images of the lesion, which can be compared with conventional histopathologic findings, and has revealed additional findings to suggest an association with sweat ducts.

Conclusion

Although the exact etiology of dyshidrotic eczema remains unknown, given the presence of metal allergy in patients with dyshidrotic eczema, and the improvement of the symptoms by removing metal allergens, metal allergy is regarded as one of the important potential etiologic factors for dyshidrotic eczema. This hypothesis is supported by previous reports of nickel-induced eczematous lesions on the palmoplantar areas, which are probably due to condensed metal allergens excreted along with sweat. Nonetheless, an association between dyshidrotic eczema and sweat ducts has not yet been established. Further studies are needed to elucidate the etiology of dyshidrotic eczema; in particular, the association among dyshidrotic eczema, metal allergy, and sweat ducts are necessary to be clarified since previous reports have shown the presence of metal allergy in patients with dyshidrotic eczema and suggested a possible association between vesicles and sweat ducts.

References

1 Veien NK: Acute and recurrent vesicular hand dermatitis. Dermatol Clin 2009;27: 337–353.
2 Storrs FJ: Acute and recurrent vesicular hand dermatitis not pompholyx or dyshidrosis. Arch Dermatol 2007;143: 1578–1580.
3 Fisher AA: Contact Dermatitis, ed 3. Philadelphia, Lea & Febiger, 1986, pp 119–130.
4 Wollina U: Pompholyx: a review of clinical features, differential diagnosis, and management. Am J Clin Dermatol 2010; 11:305–314.
5 Gullet MH, Wierzbicka E, Guillet S, et al: A 3-year causative study of pompholyx in 120 patients. Arch Dermatol 2007; 143:1504–1508.
6 Christensen OB, Möller H: External and internal exposure to the antigen in the hand eczema of nickel allergy. Contact Dermatitis 1975;1:136–141.
7 Yokozeki H, Katayama I, Nishioka K: The role of metal allergy and local hyperhidrosis in the pathogenesis of pompholyx. J Dermatol 1992;19:964–967.
8 Lee WJ, Lee DW, Kim CH, Won CH, et al: Nickel-sensitive patients with vesicular hand eczema: oral challenge with a diet naturally high in nickel. J Eur Acad Dermatol Venereol 2010;24:235–236.
9 Lee WJ, Lee DW, Kim CH, Won CH, et al: Pompholyx with bile-coloured vesicles in a patient with jaundice: are sweat ducts involved in the development of pompholyx? J Eur Acad Dermatol Venereol 2010;24:235–236.

Aya Nishizawa
Department of Dermatology
National Defense Medical College
3-2 Namiki
Tokorozawa 359-8513 (Japan)
E-Mail ayanishiza@yahoo.co.jp

Yokozeki H, Murota H, Katayama I (eds): Perspiration Research.
Curr Probl Dermatol. Basel, Karger, 2016, vol 51, pp 86–93 (DOI: 10.1159/000446786)

Pathophysiology and Treatment of Hyperhidrosis

Tomoko Fujimoto

Department of Dermatology, Graduate School of Medical and Dental Sciences, Tokyo Medical and Dental University, Tokyo, Japan

Abstract

Primary focal hyperhidrosis is a disease of unknown cause with profuse perspiration of local sites (head, face, palms, soles of feet, and axillae) that adversely affects daily life. Guidelines have been proposed in the USA [1], Canada [2], and Japan [3]. The symptoms impair quality of life, with significant negative effects on daily existence and personal relationships. The current goal in medical practice for patients with hyperhidrosis is to provide guidance and encourage coping skills for a normal daily life, as well as give appropriate advice regarding treatment options. On occasion, in order to improve quality of life, it is necessary to recommend surgical therapy when conservative treatment fails; this requires an understanding of the mechanisms of available treatments and their effects. This paper reviews theories of primary focal hyperhidrosis with regard to pathology, epidemiology, and treatment.

Concept and Pathology of Primary Focal Hyperhidrosis

Primary focal hyperhidrosis is defined as a condition in which profuse perspiration occurs on local sites such as the head, face, palms, soles, and axillae to a degree that interferes with daily life, independent of hyperthermia or mental stress. Generated sweat is derived from eccrine glands, with the basic function of thermoregulation and moisturization. Sweat also contains antimicrobial peptides and secretory IgA, and is involved in natural immunity against bacteria and viruses. Many eccrine sweat glands are distributed on the palms, with a density of about 600–700/cm^2. Others are on the forehead and axilla (360 ± 60/cm^2) and the cheek (300 ± 80/cm^2), and are the least numerous on the trunk (65 ± 20/cm^2) and extremities (120 ± 30/cm^2) [4]. However, there is no morpho-

Table 1. Causes of secondary hyperhidrosis (from Hornberger et al. [1])

Systemic
Drug-induced, drug abuse, cardiovascular disease, respiratory failure, infection, malignant tumor, endocrine metabolic diseases (hyperthyroidism, low blood sugar, pheochromocytoma, acromegaly, carcinoid tumor), neurological disorder (Parkinson's disease)
Focal
Cerebral infarction, peripheral neuropathy, compensatory sweating (cerebral infarction, spinal cord injury, neuropathy, Ross syndrome), Frey syndrome, gustatory sweating, eccrine nevus, anxiety disorder, unilateral focal hyperhidrosis (neuropathy, tumor)

logical difference between patients with primary palmar hyperhidrosis and healthy individuals regarding the number and distribution of sweat glands. Sweat glands are of two types: active sweat glands are able to secrete sweat and inactive sweat glands lack that ability. Patients with hyperhidrosis have a higher ratio of active sweat glands. However, whether the incidence of primary focal hyperhidrosis is influenced by environmental factors such as climate remains unknown. Perspiration from eccrine sweat glands at the periphery is induced by stimulation from cholinergic postganglionic sympathetic fibers, but the central mechanism has not yet been identified. However, involvement of central nervous system locations such as the amygdala, cingulate cortex, medulla, frontal lobe, hippocampus, and amygdaloid nucleus is presumed [5, 6].

Classification of Hyperhidrosis

Hyperhidrosis is classified according to the distribution (systemic or focal) and causes of perspiration (primary or secondary). The distribution of perspiration sites is determined at the initial interview and examination, and a more detailed interview is required to determine laterality or whether a proximal or distal body part is involved. Furthermore, the areas of perspiration must be confirmed objectively, as symptoms of excessive perspiration reported by a patient may in fact represent compensation for a pathological anhidrotic condition. A perspiration test is required to confirm the patient's complaint.

In secondary hyperhidrosis, the causative condition requires diagnosis and treatment. The classification of secondary hyperhidrosis [3] (table 1) requires an interview and medical examination as well as a hematological screening test for thyroid function and collagen disease at the initial visit.

Epidemiology

There have been many reports on the epidemiology of primary focal hyperhidrosis, with varying results. Palmar hyperhidrosis has a prevalence of 0.6–1% in Israel [7], 2.8% in the USA [8], and 4.36% in China [9]. The survey conducted in the USA was the largest. Of the 2.8% of the population affected by primary hyperhidrosis, 50.8% (1.4% of the entire population) have severe axillary hyperhidrosis. The mean age of affected patients is 40 years, the mean age at onset is 25 years, and prevalence peaks between 25 and 64 years of age, with the lowest prevalence in those aged 12 years or younger [8]. A survey conducted in China among students aged between 15 and 22 years in selected areas showed that the mean prevalence was 4.36%, and severe hyperhidrosis was seen in 6.21% (0.27% of the total); the mean age at onset was 12.27 ± 2.12 years, and 17.9% had a family history [9]. In 2008 in Japan, a na-

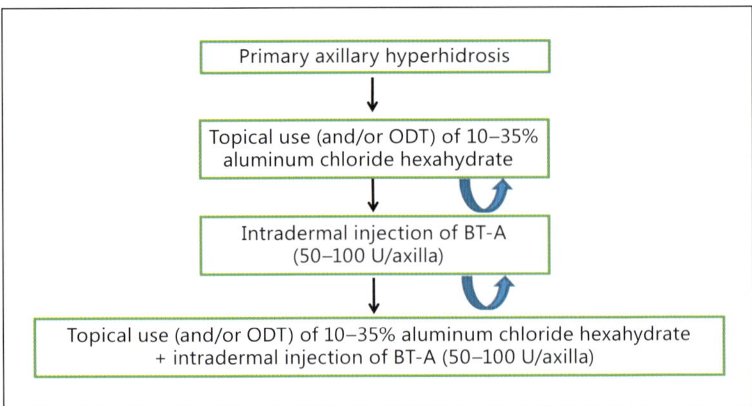

Fig. 1. Treatment algorithm for axillary hyperhidrosis. ODT = Occlusive dressing therapy.

tional survey of those aged between 5 and 65 years in selected areas showed that the prevalence of primary focal hyperhidrosis was 5.33%, with a mean age at onset of 13.8 years. The soles were involved in 2.79%, with a mean age at onset of 19.5 years, the axillae in 5.75%, with a mean age at onset of 19.5 years, and the head in 4.7%, with a mean age at onset of 21.2 years [10]. The prevalence is similar to that in a Chinese report [9]. A possible racial difference has been suggested for the prevalence of primary focal hyperhidrosis. An epidemiological survey in Hawaii reported that there were more Japanese-American patients with hyperhidrosis of the palms and soles [11], suggesting involvement of a genetic background.

Symptoms and Diagnosis

Hyperhidrosis is also classified according to whether one or more sites are involved. The amount of perspiration increases while awake, but perspiration does not occur during sleep when cortical brain activity decreases. The amount of perspiration tends to be reduced in seasons when outdoor temperature is low, and the amount of perspiration tends to increase in an environment with high temperature and high humidity; however, in severe cases, excessive perspiration is seen regardless of the season.

Hyperhidrosis of the Palms and Soles

Onset occurs during childhood or puberty. In severe cases, sweating may be so excessive that it drips off the hands and feet, which are always damp, while the fingertips may be cold with a purplish color. It is assumed that in addition to direct nerve involvement in perspiration, vasomotor nerve activity is also increased, and skin temperature decreases as a result of transpiration of sweat and vasoconstriction. In mild cases, the hands and feet may sometimes be dry, but profuse perspiration occurs temporarily when there is mental stress or when something is held in the hands. The symptoms of hyperhidrosis cause great discomfort for patients. Documents are moistened by sweat, there is discomfort with handshaking, and a personal computer and cell phone can be damaged.

Axillary Hyperhidrosis

The onset is likely to occur after axillary hair starts to grow during puberty. This is caused by mental stress and increased body temperature, and excessive perspiration with bilateral symmetry occurs in the axillae, leaving stains on underwear or shirts; patients are often forced to change

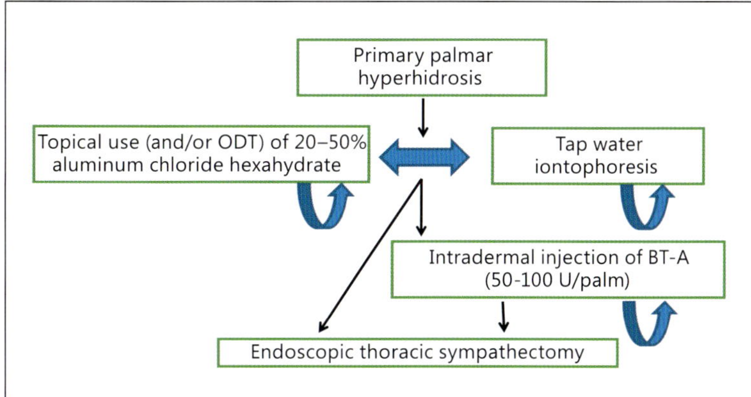

Fig. 2. Treatment algorithm for palmar hyperhidrosis.

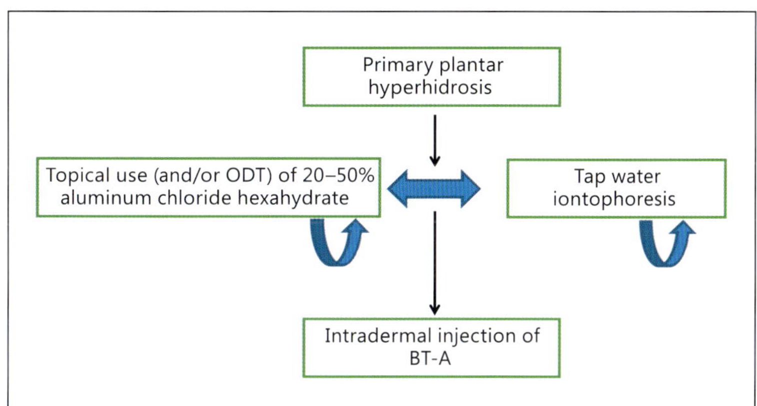

Fig. 3. Treatment algorithm for plantar hyperhidrosis.

clothes several times a day. Perspiration extends to the area beyond the axillary hair, and causes much distress in terms of personal relationships and the selection of clothes (e.g. colors and materials).

Craniofacial Hyperhidrosis
Onset is often during puberty and adolescence. Men are more likely to develop this condition. It is caused by mental stress and increased body temperature, and excessive perspiration occurs on the entire head covered by hair and on the forehead. Hair may become as wet as if a patient has taken a shower.

Treatment and Treatment Algorithms

The treatment algorithms following the diagnosis of primary focal hyperhidrosis are summarized in figures 1–4 by site. The common first choices are application of aluminum chloride or iontophoresis therapy, which are associated with fewer adverse effects. Botulinum therapy and thoracic sympathectomy (TS) also have a major role in treatment. An optional initial ancillary therapy is the use of oral anticholinergic drugs, as there is almost no other option for craniofacial hyperhidrosis.

External Use of Aluminum Chloride Solution
This is the first choice for hyperhidrosis of any site and at any age. An organic action mechanism

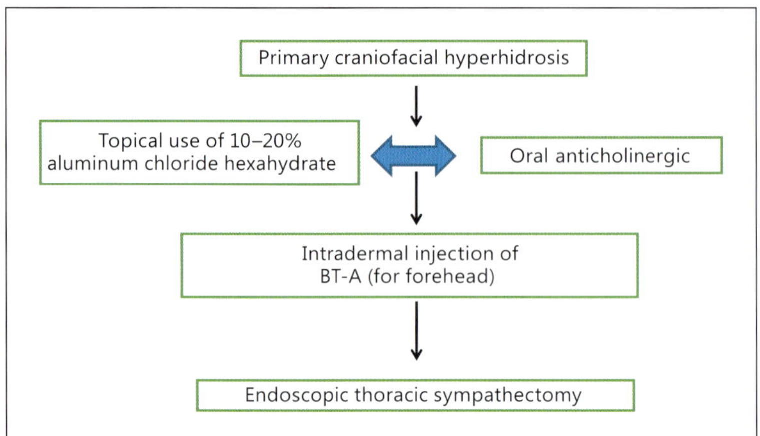

Fig. 4. Treatment algorithm for craniofacial hyperhidrosis.

is assumed: the components of aluminum chloride block exits of perspiration by binding to sweat ducts in the horny cell layer [12]. There are many highly reliable reports of efficacy, including one claiming effectiveness in a double-blind test on the palms [13]. In general, 20% aluminum chloride solution is used, but effectiveness in severe hyperhidrosis of the palms and soles has been confirmed by applying a 50% solution, or a 30% solution with adhesion to the horny cell layer enhanced by using salicylic acid petrolatum as a base, in accordance with severity [14]. Therefore, treatment can progress through improved adherence using preparations of different concentrations and formulations (table 2). Long-term safety was verified in a study on 50% aluminum chloride solution used for at least 1 year [15]. Irritant contact dermatitis was the main adverse effect, with a frequency of 45.3% during treatment of the palms, but continuous use was possible by restricting the frequency of application. Allergic contact dermatitis induced by aluminum chloride is very rare, and its safety is not problematic.

Tap Water Iontophoresis Therapy

Double-blind studies have reported that the amount of perspiration was reduced by immersing the palms and soles in tap water and supplying direct current (DC) electricity to the bath [16, 17]. The effect is reportedly due to damage and stenosis of the sweat pores caused by hydrogen ions produced when electric current is supplied [18]. In practice, a vat made of plastic is filled with tap water sufficient to cover both palms or soles, a circuit is created, and current is supplied at 10–19 mA for 10–15 min. An effect is likely to be seen following the 5th or 6th treatment on a 1- to 2-times/week basis. The number of follow-up visits is adjusted as needed. This can be used for patients in whom aluminum chloride causes irritant contact dermatitis, with similar effectiveness. Pain is caused by the electric current, and current strength is adjusted according to patient tolerance. It is suitable for palms and soles, but technically difficult to apply to the axillae, head, and face.

Local Injection of Botulinum Toxin A-Type Formulation

Botulinum neurotoxin is produced by *Clostridium botulinum*, a Gram-positive bacterium, and comprises 7 types (A to G). The highly purified botulinum toxin type A (BT-A) has superior efficacy and duration of action. It acts to inhibit acetylcholine release from the junctional mem-

Table 2. Kinds of topical aluminum chloride

Aluminum chloride	Composition		Uses of aluminum chloride
20% aluminum chloride (with or without ethanol)	Aluminum chloride hexahydrate Dehydrated ethanol Purified water Total amount	20 g 20 ml q.s. 100 ml	For all of the skin other than the mucosa; suitable for topical application with ethanol and ODT therapy without ethanol
50% aluminum chloride (with or without ethanol)	Aluminum chloride hexahydrate Dehydrated ethanol Purified water Total amount	50 g 20 ml q.s. 100 ml	For severe parts, especially palms and soles; suitable for topical application with ethanol and ODT therapy without ethanol
30% aluminum chloride with salicylic acid ointment	10% salicylic acid ointment Petrolatum Aluminum chloride hexahydrate Glycerin Total amount	157.5 g 157.5 g 135 g 75 ml 525 g	For severe parts, especially palms and soles; suitable for topical application, and ODT therapy

branes of cholinergic nerves [19]. Botox® (Allergan Inc.) and Dysport® (Ipsen) are mainly used; the potency of Botox® is reportedly 1.5–4 times higher than that of Dysport® [20, 21].

In 1996, Bushara et al. [22] first reported that BT-A was effective for axillary hyperhidrosis and subsequently it was also used for hyperhidrosis of the palms and soles. There are many reports of the highly inhibitory effect on perspiration with good evidence from double-blind randomized studies for hyperhidrosis of the palms and soles, axillae, head, and face. The problems associated with BT-A are pain at the time of injection and muscle weakness at the injection sites on the palms and forehead. In order to control pain at the time of injection, external use of local anesthetics, cooling with an ice pack, intravenous injection of anesthetics (Bier block) [23], and peripheral nerve block [24] are conducted prior to the injection. Muscle weakness in the fingers is proportional to the dose, but is mild and temporary, and lessens with observation alone [25]. The recommended doses of BT-A are Botox® 50–100 U or Dysport® 100–200 U for one hand or foot, and Botox® 50 U or Dysport® 100–200 U for one axilla. The reports on the dose of Botox® for hyperhidrosis of the head and face vary, but local injection using Botox® is recommended at a dose of up to 100 U [2].

Internal Medical Therapy

Anticholinergic Drugs. Therapy for focal hyperhidrosis using anticholinergic drugs is widely reported, but most are case reports. In a review of the evidence for nonsurgical therapy [26], anticholinergic drugs are only recommended for cases in which external therapy, iontophoresis, and Botox® are not effective. However, as hyperhidrosis of the face is difficult to treat other than by external means, the Canadian Dermatology Association [2] advises internal use of the anticholinergic drug glycopyrronium bromide (glycopyrrolate) as the first choice for moderate-to-severe hyperhidrosis of the face. There are studies in which glycopyrronium bromide [27, 28] and propantheline bromide [29, 30] were effective for focal hyperhidrosis. A randomized study was conducted in Germany on methantheline bromide, which was reportedly effective for axillary hyperhidrosis, but not hyperhidrosis of the palms and soles [31]. Anticholinergic drugs are therefore useful and may be tried as supportive treatment.

Other Therapeutic Agents. There are case reports in which clonidine hydrochloride, the benzodiazepine tofisopam, the antiepileptic agent topiramate, the selective serotonin reuptake inhibitor paroxetine with anticholinergic effects, and the tricyclic antidepressant amitriptyline were also reportedly effective for hyperhidrosis of the face. However, these reports all had a limited number of patients and lack reliability.

Psychotherapy (Mental Healing)

Psychotherapy alone cannot be effective for patients with primary focal hyperhidrosis, but cognitive and biofeedback therapy may increase efficacy by concomitant use with other conservative treatments.

Sympathectomy and Vicarious Perspiration

Shelley and Florence [32] reported that the inhibitory effects on perspiration from TS for palmar hyperhidrosis extend from the upper half of the chest to the parietal region. Thus, TS has widely been applied as treatment not only for hyperhidrosis of the palms, but also for the axillae and face. In the 1990s, endoscopic TS became popular following the introduction of thoracoscopy. Endoscopic TS almost completely stops perspiration of the palms, but compensatory hyperhidrosis (CH) occurs at high rates. However, the degree of CH is subjective, and the frequency differs among reports. Moderate or severe CH decreases patient satisfaction.

Thus, surgical treatment for hyperhidrosis should only be recommended for patients who have severe impairment of daily life. As patients are often in their late teens to 30s and have active social and personal relationships, many strongly desire surgery. However, because sympathectomy is irreversible, and some patients suffer mental distress from subsequent CH, it should only be performed on patients diagnosed with severe hyperhidrosis refractory to conservative therapy. Moreover, efficacy should be expected with blocking at a T3 or lower level, and patients should be fully informed of the risk of CH and provide written consent for treatment. Furthermore, T2 region block is necessary for perspiration of the face and head, but development of CH is almost inevitable. Therefore, it is important to weigh the risks and benefits.

Nerve Block

The number of facilities performing nerve block is limited and opinions on its value are not unified. Recently, stellate ganglion block using a laser (Super Lizer), which produces infrared radiation in the wavelength range of 0.6–1.6 μm, has been tried. Sympathetic ganglion block is less invasive than conventional sympathectomy, and can be an option prior to resection [33, 34].

Possible Novel Therapeutic Agents

Choices of treatment for hyperhidrosis are limited, often with no other option if the first treatment fails. However, anticholinergic drugs for external use and other novel drugs have been studied and developed recently. Better medical care may be available as novel treatments effective for many patients with fewer adverse effects are developed.

References

1 Hornberger J, Grimes K, Naumann M, et al: Recognition, diagnosis, and treatment of primary focal hyperhidrosis. J Am Acad Dermatol 2004;51:274–286.

2 Solish N, Bertucci V, Dansereau A, et al: A comprehensive approach to the recognition, diagnosis, and severity-based treatment of focal hyperhidrosis: recommendations of the Canadian Hyperhidrosis Advisory Committee. Dermatol Surg 2007;33:908–923.

3 Fujimoto T, Yokozeki H, Katayama I, et al: The guideline for primary focal hyperhidrosis in Japan. Jpn J Dermatol 2015;125:1379–1400.

4 Sato K, Kang WH, Saga K, Sato KT: Biology of sweat glands and their disorders. I. Normal sweat gland function. J Am Acad Dermatol 1989;20:537–563.
5 Homma S, Matsunami K, Han XY, et al: Hippocampus in relation to mental sweating response evoked by memory recall and mental calculation: a human electroencephalography study with dipole tracing. Neurosci Lett 2001;305: 1–4.
6 Asahina M, Poudel A, Hirano S: Sweating on the palm and sole: physiological and clinical relevance. Clin Auton Res 2015;25:153–159.
7 Adar R, Kurchin A, Zweig A, et al: Palmar hyperhidrosis and its surgical treatment: a report of 100 cases. Ann Surg 1977;186:34–41.
8 Strutton DR, Kowalski JW, Glaser DR, Stang PE: US prevalence of hyperhidrosis and impact on individuals with axillary hyperhidrosis: results from a national survey. J Am Acad Dermatol 2004;51:241–248.
9 Li X, Chen R, Tu YR, et al: Epidermiological survey of primary palmar hyperhidrosis in adolescents. Chin Med J 2007;120:2215–2217.
10 Fujimoto T, Kawahara K, Yokozeki H: Epidemiological study and considerations of focal hyperhidrosis in Japan: from questionnaire analysis. J Dermatol 2013;40:886–890.
11 Cloward RB: Treatment of hyperhidrosis Palmaris (sweaty hands); a familial disease in Japanese. Hawaii Med J 1957; 16:381–389.
12 Yanagishita T, Tamada Y, Ohshima Y, et al: Histological localization of aluminium in topical aluminum chloride treatment for palmar hyperhidrosis. J Dermatol Sci 2012;67:69–71.
13 Fujimoto T, Inoue R, Yokozeki H, et al: Evaluation of the efficacy of topical aluminum chloride for primary palmar hyperhidrosis in a double-blind examination. Jpn J Dermatol 2013;123:281–289.
14 Benohanian A, et al: Localized hyperhidrosis treated with aluminum chloride in a salicylic acid gel base. Int J Dermatol 1998;37:701–708.
15 Fujimoto T, Yokozeki H: Evaluation of the efficacy and side effects about a long-term use of 50% topical aluminum chloride for primary palmar hyperhidrosis. J Environ Dermatol Cutan Allergol 2015;9:238–242.
16 Dahl JC, Glent-Madsen L: Treatment of hyperhidrosis manuum by tap water iontophoresis. Acta Derm Venerol 1998; 69:346–348.
17 Yokozeki H, Ooshiro Y, Katayama I, et al: Quantitative evaluation of the effect of iontophoresis for palmoplantar hyperhidrosis. Jpn J Dermatol 1992;102: 583–586.
18 Sato K, Timm DE, Sato F, et al: Generation and transit pathway of H+ is critical for inhibition of palmar sweating by iontophoresis in water. J Appl Physiol (1985) 1993;75:2258–2264.
19 Rusciani L, Severino E, Rusciani A: Type A botulinum toxin: a new treatment for axillary and palmar hyperhidrosis. J Drugs Dermatol 2002;1:147–151.
20 Brin MF: Botulinum toxin: chemistry, pharmacology, toxicity, and immunology. Muscle Nerve Suppl 1997;6:s146–s168.
21 Shimonetta MM, Cauhepe C, Magues JP, et al: A double-blind, randomized, comparative study of Dysport vs. Botox in primary palmar hyperhidrosis. Br J Dermatol 2003;149:1041–1045.
22 Bushara KO, Park DM, Jones JC, et al: Botulinum toxin – a possible new treatment for axillary hyperhidrosis. Clin Exp Derm 1996;21:276–278.
23 Blaheta JH, Vollert B, Zuder D, et al: Intravenous regional anesthesia (Bier's block) for botulinum toxin therapy of palmar hyperhidrosis is safe and effective. Dermatol Surg 2002;28:666–672.
24 Hayton M, Stanley JK, Lowe NJ: A review of peripheral nerve blockade as local anaesthesia in the treatment of palmer hyperhidrosis. Br J Dermatol 2003;149:447–451.
25 Lowe NJ, Yamauchi PS, Lask GP, et al: Efficacy and safety of botulinum toxin type A in the treatment of palmar hyperhidrosis: a double-blind, randomized, placebo-controlled study. Dermatol Surg 2002;28:822–827.
26 Reisfeld R, Berliner KI: Evidence-based review of the nonsurgical management of hyperhidrosis. Thorac Surg Clin 2008; 18:147–166.
27 Bajaj V, Langtry JAA: Use of oral glycopyrronium bromide in hyperhidrosis. Br J Dermatol 2007;157:118–121.
28 Walling HW: Systemic therapy for primary hyperhidrosis: a retrospective study of 59 patients treated with glycopyrrolate or clonidine. J Am Acad Dermatol 2012;66:387–392.
29 Zupko AG, Prokop LD: The newer anticholinergic agents. I. Effectiveness as anhydrotics. J Am Pharmac Assoc 1954; 43:35–38.
30 Ooura I: Clinical trial study of propantheline bromide for hyperhidrosis (in Japanese). J New Remedies Clin 1955;4: 41–45.
31 Hund M, Sinkgraven R, Rzany B: Randomisierte, placebokontrollierte klinische Doppelblindstudie zur Wirksamkeit und Verträglichkeit der oralen Therapie mit Methanthelium-Bromid (Vagantin®) bei fokaler Hyperhidorose. J Dtsch Dermatol Gesellschaft 2004;2:343–349.
32 Shelley WB, Florence R: Compensatory hyperhidrosis after sympathectomy. N Engl J Med 1960;263:1056–1058.
33 Ohseto K: Efficacy of thoracic sympathetic ganglion block and prediction of complications: clinical evaluation of the anterior paratracheal and posterior paravertebral approaches in 234 patients. J Anesth 1992;6:316–331.
34 Sankstone A, Cornbleet T: Facial hyperhidrosis interruption with stellate ganglion block. JAMA 1962;179:579.

Tomoko Fujimoto, MD, PhD
Department of Dermatology
Graduate School of Medical and Dental Sciences
Tokyo Medical and Dental University
1-5-45 Yushima, Bunkyo-ku
Tokyo 113-8519 (Japan)
E-Mail tntm.derm@tmd.ac.jp

Yokozeki H, Murota H, Katayama I (eds): Perspiration Research.
Curr Probl Dermatol. Basel, Karger, 2016, vol 51, pp 94–100 (DOI: 10.1159/000446787)

New Etiology of Cholinergic Urticaria

Yoshiki Tokura

Department of Dermatology, Hamamatsu University School of Medicine, Hamamatsu, Japan

Abstract

Cholinergic urticaria (CholU) is characterized by pinpoint-sized, highly pruritic wheals occurring upon sweating. Both direct and indirect theories in the interaction of acetylcholine (ACh) with mast cells have been put forward in the sweating-associated histamine release from mast cells. In the mechanism of indirect involvement of ACh, patients are hypersensitive to sweat antigen(s) and develop wheals in response to sweat substances leaking from the syringeal ducts to the dermis, possibly by obstruction of the ducts. Some patients with CholU exhibit a positive reaction to intradermal injection of their own diluted sweat, representing 'sweat allergy (hypersensitivity)'. Regarding the direct interaction theory between ACh and mast cells, we found that CholU with anhidrosis and hypohidrosis lacks cholinergic receptor M_3 ($CHRM_3$) expression in eccrine sweat gland epithelial cells. The expression of $CHRM_3$ is completely absent in the anhidrotic areas and lowly expressed in the hypohidrotic areas. In the hypohidrotic area, where CholU occurs, it is hypothesized that ACh released from nerves cannot be completely trapped by cholinergic receptors of eccrine glands and overflows to the adjacent mast cells, leading to wheals.

Cholinergic urticaria (CholU) is a condition clinically characterized by pinpoint-sized, highly pruritic wheals (fig. 1). This unique urticaria is typically provoked by stimulation such as exercise, warmth, and emotional distress, which increases the body core temperature and promotes sweating [1, 2]. The diagnosis is thus made on the basis of typical episodes of small pinpoint wheals following exercise and sweating [3]. Since acetylcholine (ACh) is known to induce both sweating and wheals when injected intradermally, it has been considered that this perspiration-associated, syringeal orifice-coincident wheal is mediated by ACh.

The mechanisms underlying CholU remains unclear, as several controversial findings have been reported. ACh is known to induce degranulation in mast cells [4, 5]. In healthy individuals, however, ACh release from sympathetic nerves induces sweating but not wheals. Therefore, mast cells seem to be unexposed to ACh in the physiological condition. A disorder in which mast cells interact directly with ACh has recently been put forward [6] (fig. 2). Another mechanism has been

Table 1. Two types of CholU

Type	Involvement of ACh	Possible mechanism
Sweat allergy type	Indirect effect of ACh on mast cells	Obstruction of sweat duct
Depressed sweating type	Direct effect of ACh on mast cells	Depressed expression of cholinergic receptors

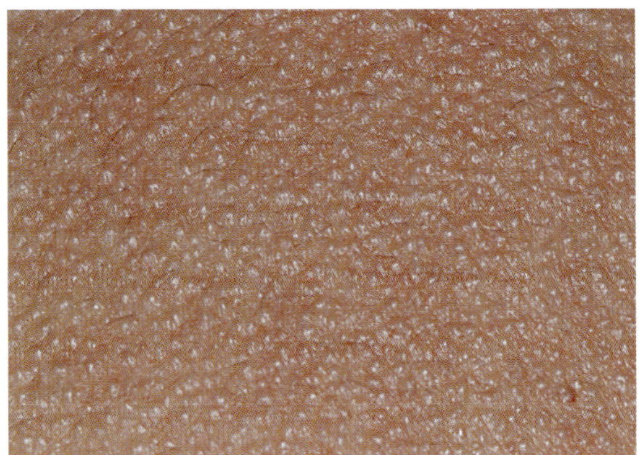

Fig. 1. Clinical appearance of CholU.

proposed. Eccrine sweat ducts are obstructed by lymphocytic inflammation around the ducts, and the resultant retention and subsequent leakage of sweat from the damaged ducts induce wheals [7]. In this theory, the direct contact of mast cells with ACh is not a requirement. ACh plays only a perspiration-promoting role, and allergy to dermally leaked sweat may evoke wheals.

This review focuses on the current understanding of the etiology of CholU with speculative mechanisms.

Clinical Tests for Cholinergic Urticaria

Intradermal injection tests with ACh and an individual patient's sweat and serum have frequently been used for the diagnosis of CholU. For the ACh injection test, 0.1 ml of 100 μg/ml ACh is intradermally injected. The development of satellite wheals around the injection site is considered as positive (fig. 3). Simultaneously, sweating around the injection site is evaluated by the iodine-starch technique. Some of the patients with CholU show a positive ACh intradermal injection test. It has been thought that the positivity vaguely represents high sensitivity to ACh, but it is rather complicated to interpret the result in relation to the mechanism.

Another skin test used for CholU study is the autologous sweat injection test. Sweat samples are usually collected from each patient's forearm after exercise, sterilized with a filter, preserved at –80°C, and diluted at 1:100 before the skin test. Samples of autologous diluted sweat (0.02 ml), and additionally autologous serum (0.05 ml), is injected intradermally into the forearm of each patient. Some of the patients show a positive result to their own sweat, representing sweat allergy (sweat hypersensitivity). There is no disease specificity since patients with atopic dermatitis also show positive results at a high frequency.

Currently, these examinations are used for classification of the subtypes of CholU or investigation of pathogenic differences in individual patients.

Sweat Allergy Type of Cholinergic Urticaria: Indirect Interaction of Acetylcholine with Mast Cells

Although the pathogenesis of CholU remains unclear, both direct and indirect theories on the interaction of ACh with mast cells have been put forward in the sweating-associated histamine release from mast cells (table 1). In the

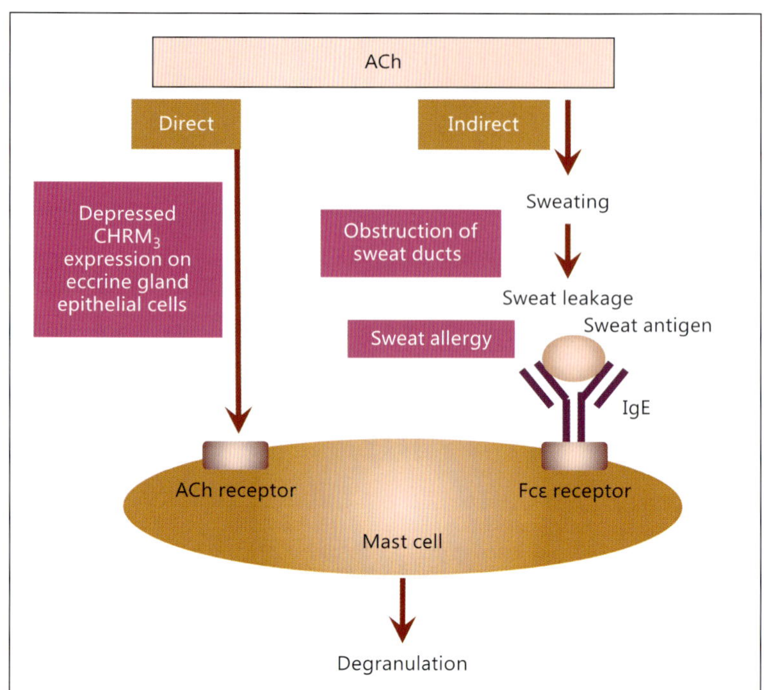

Fig. 2. Direct and indirect involvement of ACh in CholU.

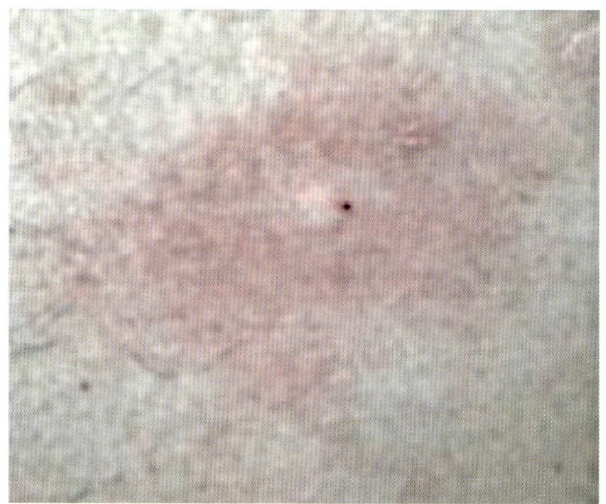

Fig. 3. Intradermal ACh injection test with satellite pinpoint wheals.

mechanism of indirect involvement of ACh, patients are hypersensitive to unknown substance(s) in their sweat and develop wheals in response to a sweat substance leaking from the syringeal ducts to the dermis, possibly by obstruction of the ducts [7, 8]. This hypothesis has been supported by the fact that some patients, but not all, with CholU exhibit a positive reaction to intradermal injection of the patient's own diluted sweat as well as ACh [9]. Thus, the ACh-indirect type is based on the 'sweat allergy (hypersensitivity)' theory. It was reported that 23 (65.7%) of 35 CholU patients associated with atopic diathesis showed basophil histamine release with semipurified sweat antigen [10]. Based on the observation that wheals are coincident with perspiration points of sweating, it is assumed that sweating causes pinpoint wheals at sweat ducts that might allow sweat to leak. However, there has been no strong evidence for sweat leakage to the dermis.

Regarding sweat antigens inducing a type I allergy, a substance derived from *Malassezia globosa* has recently been proposed [11]. MGL_1304, a major allergen in human sweat for patients with atopic dermatitis [11] and CholU [12], is secreted from *M. globosa* on human skin. Levels of serum IgE specific for purified MGL_1304 from human sweat of patients with AD and CholU were significantly higher than those of normal controls [12].

Sweat allergy is not seen in all patients with CholU. Rather, a group of CholU does not show sweat allergy. In the literature, none of the patients with CholU with anhidrosis or hypohidrosis showed positive results with intradermally injected autologous sweat, suggesting that sweat allergy is not responsible for this form of CholU, as described below.

Depressed Sweating Type of Cholinergic Urticaria: Direct Interaction of Acetylcholine with Mast Cells

Although its ability is controversial, ACh is known to induce degranulation in mast cells [4, 5]. We cultured mast cell line LAD2 cells with varying concentrations of ACh, and the degree of degranulation was measured. The addition of ACh at 10^{-5} M or more induced degranulation at a significantly higher level, and 10^{-4} M ACh exerted the maximal effect in this system [6]. It is thus assumed that ACh is capable of inducing mast cell degranulation in clinical settings where nerves, the source of ACh, are located in the vicinity.

CholU is occasionally associated with depressed perspiration, as reported under the name of anhidrosis (complete lack of sweating) or hypohidrosis (incomplete lack of sweating) [13]. From a neurological point of view, this condition is termed 'acquired idiopathic generalized anhidrosis' or more specifically 'idiopathic pure sudomotor failure' [14] accompanied by CholU. The four limbs, especially their distal portions, and the face may be the predilections of anhidrosis, which are seen in a large mosaic pattern. Sweating is usually kept in the palms and soles. In analyzing 29 reported cases of CholU with anhidrosis and/or hypohidrosis (CUAH), it is notable that 26 patients were Japanese [6]. In addition, 2 Japanese patients also had episodes of seizures upon occurrence of urticaria with or without abnormalities in electroencephalography [15, 16]. Given that ACh mediates epileptic seizures [17], convulsion possibly occurs when corticosteroid therapy induces the reexpression of ACh receptors in the brain.

In patients with CUAH, the skin surface can be divided into anhidrotic and hypohidrotic areas. For example, the anhidrotic areas typically include the four extremities and back, and the shoulders and chest are hypohidrotic areas. The patients develop pinpoint wheals on the hypohidrotic areas, but not on the anhidrotic areas. Whereas ACh injection induces no reaction at the anhidrotic site, it can yield wheals on the hypohidrotic area. ACh injection at the hypohidrotic site also may induce sweating.

The cholinergic receptor mediates wheal development [18–20]. It was demonstrated by a binding assay that muscarinic ACh receptors are reduced in the skin of patients with CholU [21]. We found that CUAH lacks cholinergic receptor M_3 ($CHRM_3$) expression in eccrine sweat gland epithelial cells [6]. The expression of $CHRM_3$ is completely absent in the anhidrotic areas, while it is incompletely decreased in the hypohidrotic areas. In addition to the depressed expression of $CHRM_3$, a disordered release of ACh esterase (AChE), a processing enzyme of ACh, may contribute to the pathogenesis of CholU [22]. The expression of AChE as well as $CHRM_3$ is lowest in CUHA and moderately abrogated in CholU [23].

Mast cells are only present in the vicinity of eccrine glands. In the anhidrotic area, mast cells do not express the $CHRM_3$, but the expression is

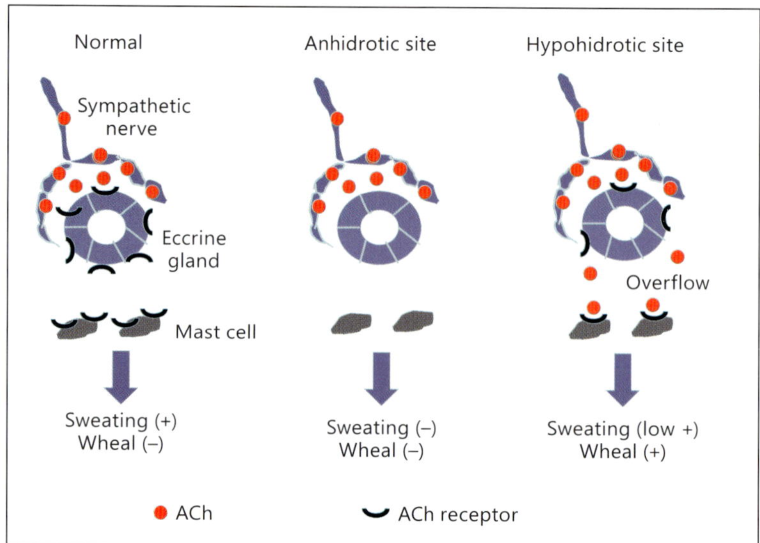

Fig. 4. Mechanism of wheals in CUAH with anhidrosis and hypohidrosis.

retained in the hypohidrotic area. Therefore, mast cells share the pattern of $CHRM_3$ expression with the eccrine gland epithelial cells in the anhidrotic and hypohidrotic areas. In the anhidrotic area, neither eccrine gland epithelial cells nor mast cells express $CHRM_3$, and it is thus reasonable that sweating and wheal formation are absent in this area. In the hypohidrotic area, it is tempting to speculate that ACh released from nerves upon exercise cannot be completely trapped by cholinergic receptors of eccrine glands and overflows to the adjacent mast cells (fig. 4). In this scenario, it is assumed that mast cells can produce histamine in response to ACh because mast cells in the hypohidrotic area express some degree of $CHRM_3$.

The injection of autologous sweat or serum does not produce positive reactions in either the hypohidrotic or anhidrotic area, suggesting the absence of sweat allergy [6, 24]. In addition, the autoimmune mechanism by autoantibodies to Fcε receptors or IgE on mast cells, as demonstrated in ordinary urticaria [25], is negated with the serum injection test.

Inflammatory Cell Infiltration around Eccrine Sweat Glands in Cholinergic Urticaria

There have been a considerable number of reports demonstrating that T lymphocytes infiltrate around eccrine sweat glands in CholU patients. Significantly higher numbers of lymphocytes and mast cells infiltrate around eccrine glands in CUHA patients than in healthy subjects or CholU patients [6, 23]. Periglandular infiltrate in CUAH patients consists of a mixture of $CD4^+$ and $CD8^+$ T cells and a mixture of $CXCR3^+$ (mostly Th1 cells) and $CCR4^+$ T cells (mostly Th2 cells) [23]. Two possible consequences may be led by the infiltrate: (1) obstruction of sweat ducts and resultant dermal leakage of sweat, and (2) reduction of $CHRM_3$ expression on sweat gland epithelial cells. Both conditions are considered to induce low perspiration and CholU. In CUAH, however, the inflammatory change unlikely induces the obstruction of sweat ducts and anhidrosis since the patients usually have no sweat allergy and develop no wheals in the anhidrotic area. The number of infiltrating lymphocytes in eccrine glands inversely correlates with the expression levels of

$CHRM_3$ and AChE. It is likely that the overproduced ACh is incapable of binding to $CHRM_3$, whose expression is reduced in eccrine glands, and may overflow to adjacent mast cells, leading to degranulation.

Since the expressions of CCL2/MCP-1, CCL5/RANTES, and CCL17/TARC are increased in the eccrine gland epithelial cells of CUHA, it is likely that T cells are attracted by these chemokines and may affect the $CHRM_3$ and AChE expression levels [23]. CholU is frequently associated with atopic conditions, especially atopic dermatitis [26], suggesting that a Th2-skewing condition might be dominant in CUHA or CholU patients. A review article showed that 43% cases of acquired idiopathic generalized anhidrosis displayed elevated serum IgE levels, suggesting an allergic etiology in CUHA [14]. Atopic dermatitis lesional skin expresses CCL2/MCP-1, CCL5/RANTES, and CCL17/TARC at remarkably higher levels than psoriatic lesions and healthy control skin [23]. $CD4^+$ and $CD8^+$ T cell populations chemoattracted by CCL2/MCP-1, CCL5/RANTES, and CCL17/TARC might affect eccrine gland epithelial cells to abrogate the expression of $CHRM_3$. It appears that mast cells also infiltrate around eccrine glands by virtue of the chemokines and promote the urticarial condition. CCL2/MCP-1, CCL5/RANTES, and CCL17/TARC have been shown to be chemoattractants for mast cells [27, 28]. These findings support the notion that CCL2/MCP-1, CCL5/RANTES, and CCL17/TARC play a crucial role in CUHA and CholU patients.

Conclusion

This chapter proposes two types of CholU: sweat allergy type and depressed sweating type [29]. Although some modification would be necessary, I believe that this categorization is helpful for better understanding CholU. One of the first-line treatments of CUAH is pulse therapy with a high dose of corticosteroids. This systemic therapy improves urticaria as well as perspiration [14]. Corticosteroids inhibit the expression of CCL2/MCP-1, CCL5/RANTES, and CCL17/TARC [30]. The treatment may decrease the downmodulatory effects of lymphocytic infiltrate on $CHRM_3$ expression and allow $CHRM_3$ to reexpress.

References

1 Moore-Robinson M, Warin RP: Some clinical aspects of cholinergic urticaria. Br J Dermatol 1968;80:794–799.

2 Hirschmann JV, Lawlor F, English JS, et al: Cholinergic urticaria. A clinical and histologic study. Arch Dermatol 1987;123:462–467.

3 Black AK, Lawlor F, Greaves MW: Consensus meeting on the definition of physical urticarias and urticarial vasculitis. Clin Exp Dermatol 1996;21:424–426.

4 Fantozzi R, Masini E, Blandina P, et al: Release of histamine from rat mast cells by acetylcholine. Nature 1978;273:473–474.

5 Blandina P, Fantozzi R, Mannaioni PF, Masini E: Characteristics of histamine release evoked by acetylcholine in isolated rat mast cells. J Physiol 1980;301:281–293.

6 Sawada Y, Nakamura M, Bito T, Fukamachi S, Kabashima R, Sugita K, Hino R, Tokura Y: Cholinergic urticaria: studies on the muscarinic cholinergic receptor M_3 in anhidrotic and hypohidrotic skin. J Invest Dermatol 2010;130:2683–2686.

7 Adachi J, Aoki T, Yamatodani A: Demonstration of sweat allergy in cholinergic urticaria. J Dermatol Sci 1994;7:142–149.

8 Kobayashi H, Aiba S, Yamagishi T, et al: Cholinergic urticaria, a new pathogenic concept: hypohidrosis due to interference with the delivery of sweat to the skin. Dermatology 2002;204:173–178.

9 Fukunaga A, Bito T, Tsuru K, et al: Responsiveness to autologous sweat and serum in cholinergic urticaria classifies its clinical subtypes. J Allergy Clin Immunol 2005;116:397–402.

10 Takahagi S, Tanaka T, Ishii K, et al: Sweat antigen induces histamine release from basophils of patients with cholinergic urticaria associated with atopic diathesis. Br J Dermatol 2009;160:426–428.

11 Hiragun T, Ishii K, Hiragun M, et al: Fungal protein MGL_1304 in sweat is an allergen for atopic dermatitis patients. J Allergy Clin Immunol 2013;132:608–615.

12 Hiragun M, Hiragun T, Ishii K, et al: Elevated serum IgE against MGL_1304 in patients with atopic dermatitis and cholinergic urticaria. Allergol Int 2014;63:83–93.

13 Itakura E, Urabe K, Yasumoto S, Nakayama J, Furue M: Cholinergic urticaria associated with acquired generalized hypohidrosis: report of a case and review of the literature. Br J Dermatol 2000;143:1064–1066.

14 Nakazato Y, Tamura N, Ohkuma A, Yoshimaru K, Shimazu K: Idiopathic pure sudomotor failure: anhidrosis due to deficits in cholinergic transmission. Neurology 2004;63:1476–1480.
15 Harada T, Yamamura Y, Ishizaki F, et al: A case of cholinergic urticaria with epileptic seizure and abnormalities on electroencephalogram (in Japanese). No To Shinkei 2001;53:863–868.
16 Takezaki S, Suzuki D, Kida K, et al: A case of cholinergic urticaria with epileptic seizure and abnormalities on electroencephalogram. J Obihiro Kosei General Hospital 2003;6:145–147.
17 Whalley BJ, Postlethwaite M, Constanti A: Further characterization of muscarinic agonist-induced epileptiform bursting activity in immature rat piriform cortex, in vitro. Neuroscience 2005;134:549–566.
18 Tong LJ, Balakrishnan G, Kochan JP, Kinét JP, Kaplan AP: Assessment of autoimmunity in patients with chronic urticaria. J Allergy Clin Immunol 1997; 99:461–465.
19 Shelly WB, Shelly ED, Ho AK: Cholinergic urticaria: acetylcholine-receptor-dependent immediate-type hypersensitivity reaction to copper. Lancet 1983;16: 843–846.
20 Baron B, Schreiber G, Sokolovsky M: Cholinergic urticaria, copper-induced hypersensitivity, and muscarinic receptor. Lancet 1983;2:55.
21 Haustein UF, Schliebs R, Schaller J: Changes in muscarinic acetylcholine receptor binding in skin slices of cholinergic urticaria. Acta Derm Venereol 1990;70:2.
22 Magnus IA, Thompson RH: Cholinesterase levels in the skin in cholinogenic urticaria and pruritus. Br J Dermatol 1956;68:283–289.
23 Sawada Y, Nakamura M, Bito T, Sakabe J, Kabashima-Kubo R, Hino R, Kobayashi M, Tokura Y: Decreased expression of acetylcholine esterase in cholinergic urticaria with hypohidrosis or anhidrosis. J Invest Dermatol 2014;134:276–279.
24 Tsuchiya T, Aoyama K, Hasegawa M, Tamura A, Ishikawa O: Cholinergic urticaria associated with hypohidrosis improved after admission. Jpn J Clin Dermatol 2004;58:129–131.
25 Hide M, Francis DM, Grattan CE, et al: Autoantibodies against the high-affinity IgE receptor as a cause of histamine release in chronic urticaria. N Engl J Med 1993;328:1599–1604.
26 Takahagi S, Tanaka T, Ishii K, et al: Sweat antigen induces histamine release from basophils of patients with cholinergic urticaria associated with atopic diathesis. Br J Dermatol 2008;160:426–428.
27 Conti P, Pang X, Boucher W, et al: Impact of Rantes and MCP-1 chemokines on in vivo basophilic cell recruitment in rat skin injection model and their role in modifying the protein and mRNA levels for histidine decarboxylase. Blood 1997; 89:4120–4127.
28 Tsunemi Y, Saeki H, Nakamura K, et al: CCL17 transgenic mice show an enhanced Th2-type response to both allergic and non-allergic stimuli. Eur J Immunol 2006;36:2116–2127.
29 Bito T, Sawada Y, Tokura Y: Pathogenesis of cholinergic urticaria in relation to sweating. Allergol Int 2012;61:539–544.
30 Hoshino M, Nakagawa T, Sano Y, et al: Effect of inhaled corticosteroid on an immunoreactive thymus and activation-regulated chemokine expression in the bronchial biopsies from asthmatics. Allergy 2005;60:317–322.

Yoshiki Tokura, MD, PhD
Department of Dermatology
Hamamatsu University School of Medicine
Handayama 1-20-1, Higashi-ku
Hamamatsu 431-3192 (Japan)
E-Mail tokura@hama-med.ac.jp

Yokozeki H, Murota H, Katayama I (eds): Perspiration Research.
Curr Probl Dermatol. Basel, Karger, 2016, vol 51, pp 101–108 (DOI: 10.1159/000446788)

Sweat Allergy

Takaaki Hiragun • Michihiro Hide

Department of Dermatology, Integrated Health Sciences, Institute of Biomedical and Health Sciences, Hiroshima University, Hiroshima, Japan

Abstract

For many years, sweat has been recognized as an exacerbation factor in all age groups of atopic dermatitis (AD) and a trigger of cholinergic urticaria (CholU). Recently, we reported the improvement of AD symptoms by spray with tannic acid, which suppresses basophil histamine release by semipurified sweat antigens in vitro, and showering that removes antigens in sweat from the skin surface. We finally identified MGL_1304 secreted by *Malassezia globosa* as a major histamine-releasing antigen in human sweat. MGL_1304 is detected as a 17-kDa protein in sweat and exhibits almost the highest histamine-release ability from basophils of patients with AD and CholU among antigens derived from *Malassezia* species. Moreover, serum levels of anti-MGL_1304 IgE of patients with AD and CholU were significantly higher than those of normal controls. Desensitization therapy using autologous sweat or MGL_1304 purified from culture of *M. globosa* or its cognates might be beneficial for patients with intractable CholU due to sweat allergy.

Background of Sweat Allergy

Atopic dermatitis (AD) is a chronic relapsing eczematous skin disease characterized by pruritus and inflammation, accompanied by cutaneous physiological dysfunction (dry and barrier-disrupted skin) [1]. Sweat is considered as one of the major exacerbation factors for AD across all age groups [2]. It might be due to the distribution of eczematous lesions in sweat-susceptible areas (such as cubital and popliteal fossa). Cholinergic urticaria (CholU) is a subtype of chronic inducible urticarias, symptoms of which are evoked by sweating due to the elevation of body core temperature [3]. Although the pathogenesis of CholU has not been fully clarified, approximately half of the patients with CholU are known to possess atopic diathesis [4].

Nakamizo et al. [5] proposed that CholU be categorized into four subtypes based on its pathogenesis: (1) CholU with poral occlusion, (2) CholU with acquired generalized hypohidrosis, (3) CholU with sweat allergy, and (4) idiopathic

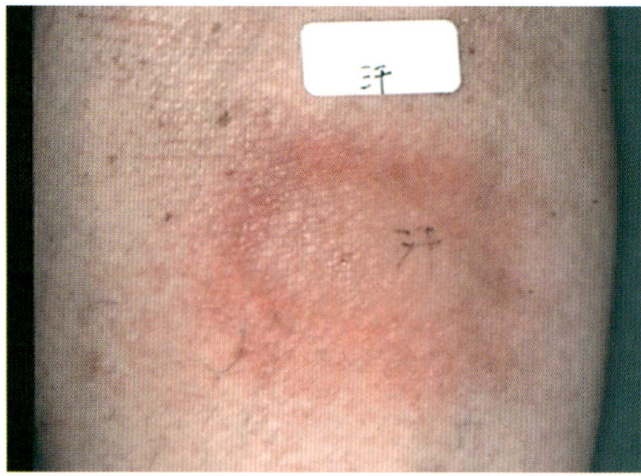

Fig. 1. Positive reaction of an intradermal skin test using autologous sweat in a patient with AD.

Table 1. Positive rates of sweat allergy in patients with AD and CholU

First author	AD	CholU	Healthy controls
Adachi [6]	96 (43/45)	–	18 (4/22)
Adachi [7]	–	100 (20/20)	0 (0/20)
Hide [8]	85 (56/66)	–	11 (3/27)
Tanaka [9]	77 (47/61)	–	9 (4/46)
Takahagi [4]	–	66 (23/35)	0 (0/14)

Values represent % (n/n).

CholU. Sweat allergy, hypersensitivity against one's own sweat, was first described by Adachi and Aoki [6] in 1989. They demonstrated hypersensitivity against sweat in patients with AD [6] and subsequently CholU [7] by performing intradermal skin tests with autologous sweat. A representative positive reaction of an intradermal skin test with autologous sweat is shown in figure 1. In 2002, Hide et al. [8] reported that patients with AD possessed hypersensitivity against crude and semipurified sweat by performing intradermal skin tests and basophil histamine release tests (HRTs). We further purified human sweat from healthy volunteers by histamine-releasing activity of basophils obtained from patients with AD, and demonstrated that histamine release induced by the semipurified sweat antigen is dependent on specific IgE in the sera of patients with AD [9].

These observations have proven sweat allergy as a type I hypersensitivity against crude sweat or ingredients in sweat. The positive rates of sweat allergy in AD and CholU were 77–96% and 66–100%, respectively, as shown in table 1. The antigen lost its histamine-releasing activity following treatment with proteinase K or trypsin [9], suggesting that the antigen in sweat was protein. The sera of patients with positive HRTs against semipurified sweat antigen also possessed histamine-release neutralization activity due to either IgE and/or IgG antibody against sweat antigen [10]. However, the substance which induces histamine release from basophils of patients with AD and CholU had not been identified for more than two decades since the first report by Adachi and Aoki [6].

Human eccrine sweat consists of water, sodium, potassium, bicarbonate, chloride, lactate, urea, ammonia, small quantities of various amino acids, and proteins [11]. Proteins in eccrine sweat consist of proteases (e.g. kallikreins), protease inhibitors (e.g. cystatins), and antimicrobial peptides (e.g. dermcidin). Besides substances that induce the immediate hypersensitivity reaction, proinflammatory cytokines (IL-1α, IL-1β, and IL-31) are contained in human sweat [12]. It is also reported that the concentration of nickel in sweat [13] and serum [14] is higher in patients with intrinsic AD than in patients with extrinsic AD. Moreover, the positive rate of patch testing to nickel and cobalt in intrinsic AD is high. Thus, nickel excreted in sweat might be an exacerbation factor for intrinsic AD.

Identification of MGL_1304 as a Sweat Antigen

A certain population of patients with AD show IgE reactivity to a variety of human protein antigens, namely autoallergy [15]. Although the path-

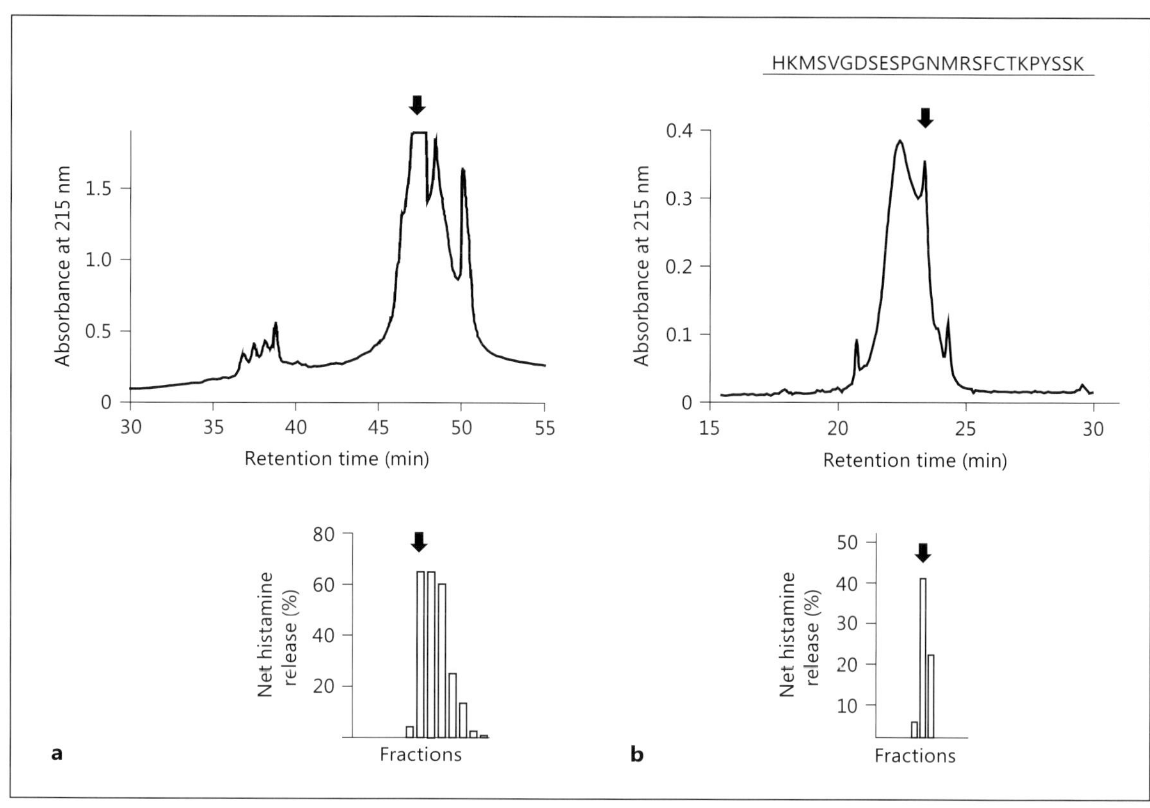

Fig. 2. Identification of MGL_1304 in human sweat. The semipurified sweat antigen (QRX) was purified with an Aqua 5 µm-C18-200 Å (**a**) and with a Jupiter 5 µm-C18-300 Å HPLC column (**b**) based on histamine-releasing activity (bars in lower panels). The fraction indicated by arrows in **a** was further purified in **b**. The peptide sequence identified by mass spectrometry is shown in **b**. From Hiragun et al. [21] with permission.

ological roles of such autoantigens in AD are still controversial, some of them have cross antigenicities to environmental allergens derived from pollen or fungi [16, 17]. Among them, human manganese superoxide dismutase and thioredoxin were highly cross-reactive to the counterparts of *Malassezia sympodialis*, Mala s 11 and Mala s 13, respectively, suggesting pathogenic roles of the autoallergy in AD [18, 19]. On the other hand, a recent report showed that the intensity of IgE autoreactivity, but not IgE against exogenous allergens, seemed to follow skin inflammation, suggesting that autoallergy was a mirror of tissue damage [20]. We hypothesized that sweat antigens are of human origin and generated a cDNA library from mRNA of human skin. We initially tried the expression cloning of sweat antigens and examined 120,000 cDNA clones by HRTs. However, no cDNA clone that induced histamine release from basophils of patients with AD was detected (unpublished).

Meanwhile, we further purified the semipurified sweat antigen (QRX) [9] with two additional reverse-phase chromatography columns (fig. 2). Mass spectrometric analysis of a peak fraction of UV absorption, which corresponded to the peak fraction of histamine-releasing activity revealed a sequence identical to a part of the hypothetical protein secreted by *Malassezia globosa*, MGL_1304 [21]. We then generated recombinant MGL_1304 by *Escherichia coli*, and confirmed that it induces histamine release from basophils from patients with AD. The recombinant MGL_1304 was immunologically identical with previously reported [9] 'semipurified sweat antigen' by neutralization assays using immunoblotting and degranulation assays with RBL-48 cells. Immunoblots with monoclonal antibody against MGL_1304 revealed that the size of MGL_1304 was 17 and 29 kDa, respectively, in sweat and in *M. globosa* (fig. 3). These observations indicated that MGL_1304 secreted by *M. globosa* was processed by unidentified proteases and turned into the mature form in sweat.

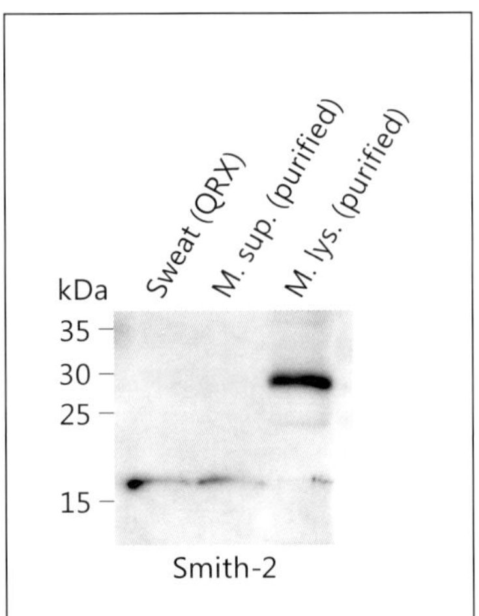

Fig. 3. An immunoblot of MGL_1304. MGL_1304 was cleaved and secreted into sweat from *M. globosa*. Histamine-releasing activity was purified from sweat (QRX), culture supernatants [M. sup. (purified)], and lysates [M. lys. (purified)] of *M. globosa*. The purified proteins were blotted with Smith-2. From Hiragun et al. [21] with permission.

Establishment of an ELISA System Measuring MGL_1304-Specific Immunoglobulins

HRTs require fresh blood cells from patients. Moreover, the results are qualitative rather than quantitative. Thus, we established an ELISA system using human sera measuring immunoglobulins (IgE, IgG, and IgG4) that are specific against MGL_1304 [22]. Levels of MGL_1304-specific IgE of patients with AD and CholU were significantly higher than those of normal controls (fig. 4a). Unlike MGL_1304-specific IgE, the levels of MGL_1304-specific IgG and IgG4 of patients with AD were not significantly higher than that of normal controls. These results indicated that the sensitization of MGL_1304 occurred even in healthy individuals, and the disturbance of skin barrier function did not affect the sensitization of MGL_1304 itself. The difference might be due to atopic diathesis which tends to generate high amounts of IgE as compared with healthy individuals. The levels of IgE against MGL_1304 correlated with disease severity of AD (fig. 4b). Using human IgE monoclonal antibody that specifically binds to MGL_1304 (ABS-IgE), 1 unit of anti-MGL_1304 IgE shown in fig. 4 has been determined as 32 pg [23]. The amount of MGL_1304 in human sweat can also be measured by sandwich ELISA using ABS-IgE [23].

Generation of Recombinant MGL_1304 by *Pichia pastoris*

To estimate hypersensitivity against sweat, HRTs by purified antigen from sweat have become commercially available in Japan. However, purifying antigen from crude sweat is costly and time consuming. Recombinant MGL_1304 produced by *E. coli* had a large chaperone protein to be solubilized and lacked fungal-type glycosylation. Therefore, we generated recombinant MGL_1304 by using *P. pastoris* as a substitution of native MGL_1304 [24]. MGL_1304 by *P. pastoris* has a 100-fold higher histamine-release ability than that by *E. coli* in HRTs. Moreover, in degranula-

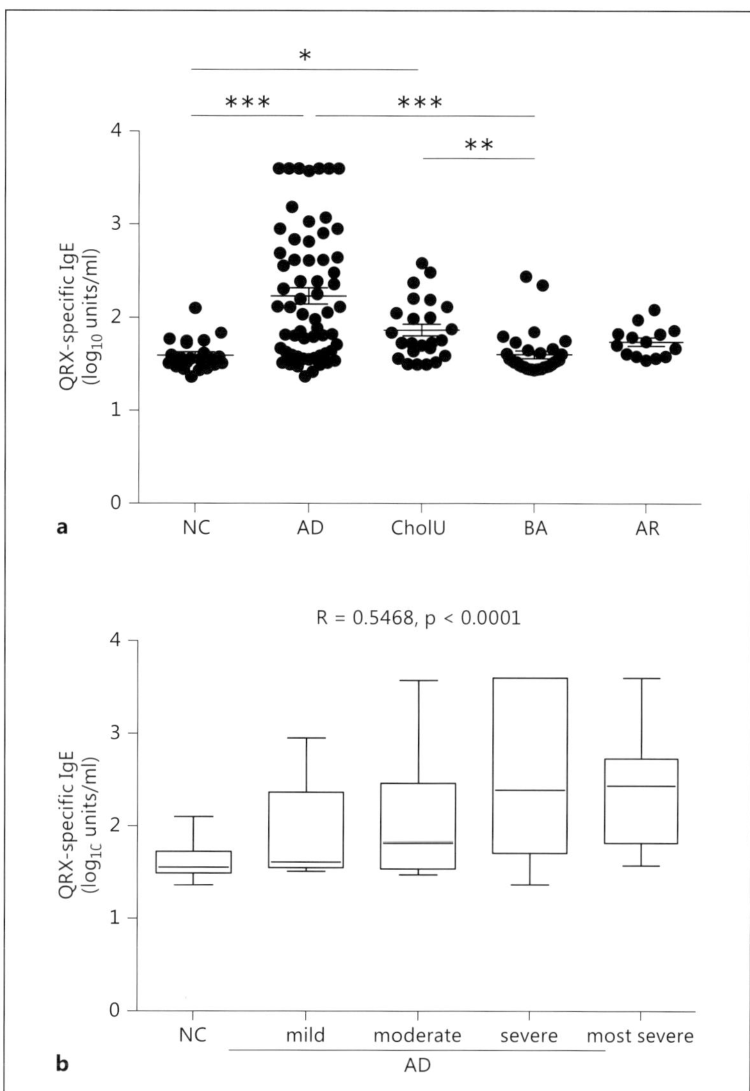

Fig. 4. Comparisons of serum levels of the semipurified sweat antigen (QRX)-specific IgE among diseases and correlations with severities of AD. Serum levels of QRX-specific IgE in patients with each disease were plotted and analyzed by the Kruskal Wallis test. The serum levels of QRX-specific IgE in patients showing various severities of AD were plotted and analyzed by Spearman's rank correlation. NC = Normal controls; BA = bronchial asthma; AR = allergic rhinitis. * $p < 0.05$, ** $p < 0.01$, *** $p < 0.001$. From Hiragun et al. [22] with permission

tion assays using RBL48 cells sensitized with sera of patients, recombinant MGL_1304 by *P. pastoris*, but not that by *E. coli*, induced release of β-hexasominidase as native antigen (fig. 5). Thus, the recombinant protein generated by *P. pastoris* may be a superior surrogate of native MGL_1304 to estimate sweat allergy.

How to Deal with Sweat Allergy

Removal of antigens from the skin surface by showering or bathing is an easy and convenient way to deal with sweat allergy in patients with AD. Kameyoshi et al. [25] and Mochizuki et al. [26] reported previously that elementary school children with AD who showered at the school during the summer season improved skin symp-

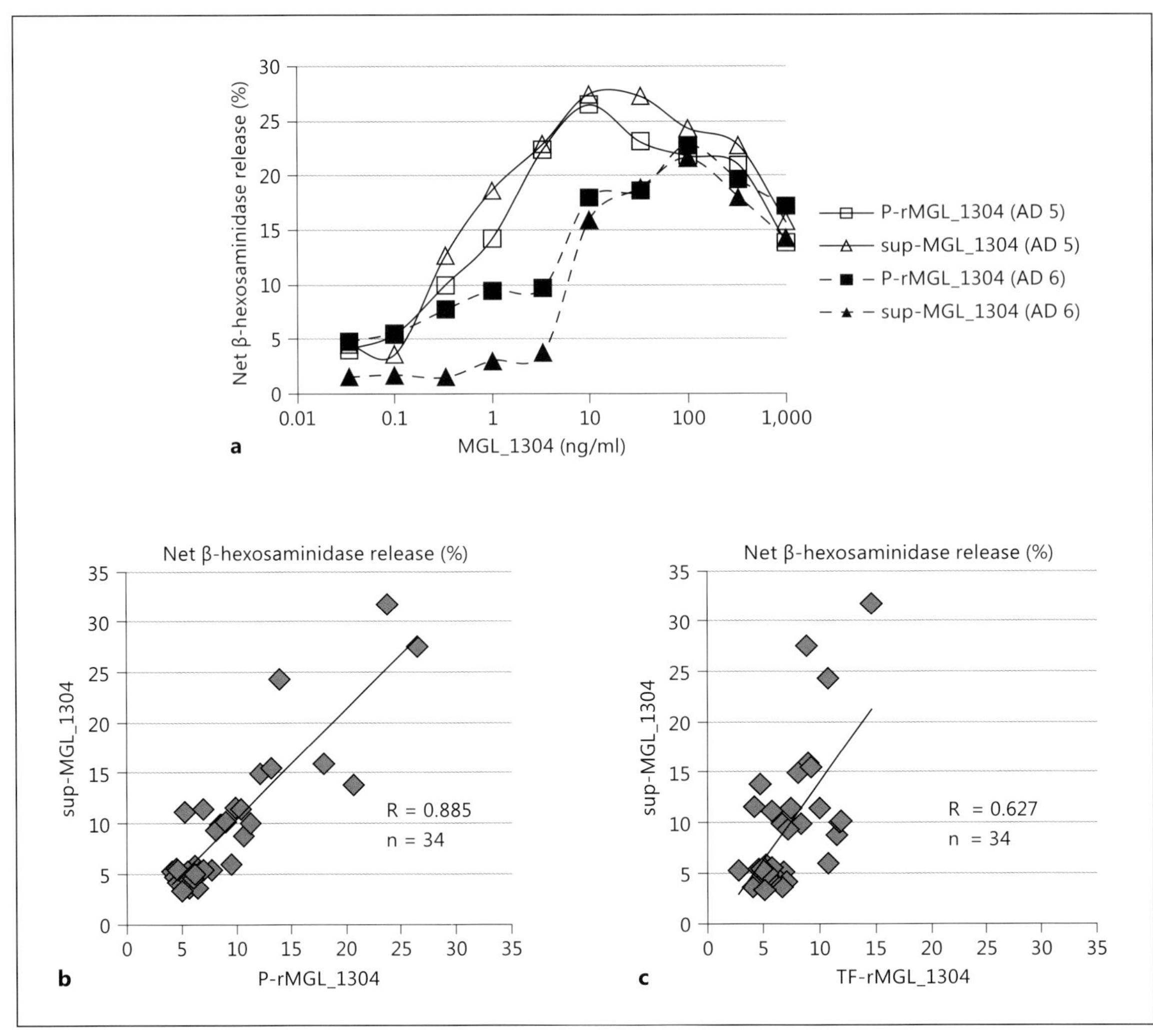

Fig. 5. Comparison of native and recombinant MGL_1304. **a** RBL-48 (cells were sensitized with 2 patients with AD, stimulated with a series of concentrations of *P. pastoris*-derived rMGL_1304 (P-rMGL_1304) and native MGL_1304 (sup-MGL_1304), and net β-hexosaminidase release (%) were measured. The concentrations of MGL_1304 were normalized by sandwich ELISA. **b** RBL-48 cells were sensitized with sera of patients with AD, stimulated with 10 ng/ml of P-rMGL_1304, 10 ng/ml of sup-MGL_1304, or 1 μg/ml of *E. coli*-derived rMGL_1304 (TF-rMGL_1304), and release of β-hexosaminidase were measured. The correlation coefficient of net β-hexosaminidase release (%) between sup-MGL_1304 and P-rMGL_1304, or sup-MGL_1304 and TF-rMGL1304 are shown. From Kan et al. [24] with permission.

toms of AD. We further explored natural substances that are harmless to human skin and neutralize the histamine-release ability of semipurified sweat allergen. We selected tannic acid (TA), a natural polyphenolic compound and protein-denaturing agent contained in grapes and green tea. Previous reports have shown that TA removed peanut antigens [27] and reduced mite allergens, but not cat allergens [28]. TA suppressed histamine release by semipurified sweat antigen

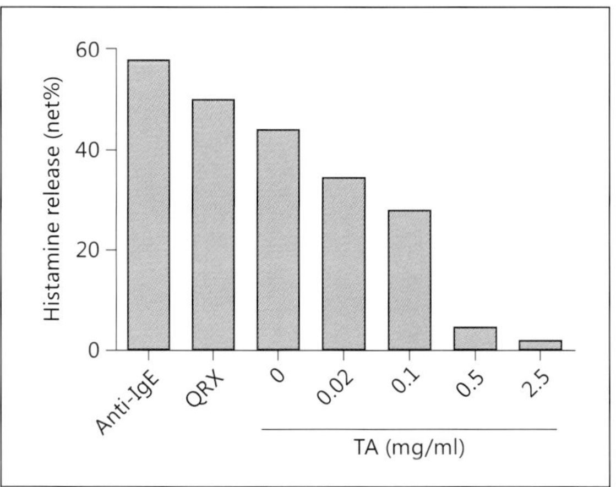

Fig. 6. Treatment with tannic acid (TA) on histamine-release activity of semipurified sweat antigen (QRX). Histamine-release activity was suppressed by TA in a concentration-dependent manner. From Shindo et al. [29] with permission.

in a dose-dependent manner in vitro (fig. 6) [29]. Spray, after bathing water, and aerosol spray containing TA all improved the symptoms of patients with AD [29]. The mechanism of the antigen-inactivating effect of TA might be degenerating and/or transferring antigens from soluble fractions into insoluble fractions [27]. In addition, TA ameliorated the inflammation of keratinocytes due to upregulation of peroxisome proliferator-activated receptor-γ [30]. Therefore, the clinical effects of TA might also be due to the effect on keratinocytes. For patients with CholU, desensitization therapy might be beneficial for those who have hypersensitivity against sweat. Kozaru et al. [31] and Tanaka et al. [32] previously reported the effect of desensitization therapy with crude sweat and semipurified sweat antigen, respectively.

Conclusions

MGL_1304 was found as a main antigen in human sweat, which induces histamine release from basophils of patients with AD. However, several questions have been left unsolved. How does MGL_1304 penetrate the epidermis and reach dermal mast cells bearing specific IgE? What are the roles of other substances in human sweat that induce histamine release? Are there any autoantigens in sweat? Further investigations are needed to understand sweat allergy and to develop better therapies for allergic diseases associated with sweat, such as AD and CholU.

References

1 Saeki H, Furue M, Furukawa F, Hide M, Ohtsuki M, Katayama I, Sasaki R, Suto H, Takehara K; Committee for Guidelines for the Management of Atopic Dermatitis of Japanese Dermatological Association: Guidelines for management of atopic dermatitis. J Dermatol 2009;36:563–577.

2 Katayama I, Kohno Y, Akiyama K, Aihara M, Kondo N, Saeki H, Shoji S, Yamada H, Nakamura K; Japanese Society of Allergology: Japanese guideline for atopic dermatitis 2014. Allergol Int 2014;63:377–398.

3 Magerl M, Borzova E, Giménez-Arnau A, Grattan CE, Lawlor F, Mathelier-Fusade P, Metz M, Młynek A, Maurer M: The definition and diagnostic testing of physical and cholinergic urticarias – EAACI/GA^{2}LEN/EDF/UNEV consensus panel recommendations. Allergy 2009;64:1715–1721.

4 Takahagi S, Tanaka T, Ishii K, Suzuki H, Kameyoshi Y, Shindo H, Hide M: Sweat antigen induces histamine release from basophils of patients with cholinergic urticaria associated with atopic diathesis. Br J Dermatol 2009;160:426–428.

5 Nakamizo S, Egawa G, Miyachi Y, Kabashima K: Cholinergic urticaria: pathogenesis-based categorization and its treatment options. J Eur Acad Dermatol Venereol 2012;26:114–116.

6 Adachi K, Aoki T: IgE antibody to sweat in atopic dermatitis. Acta Derm Venereol Suppl (Stockh) 1989;144:83–87.

7 Adachi J, Aoki T, Yamatodani A: Demonstration of sweat allergy in cholinergic urticaria. J Dermatol Sci 1994;7:142–149.

8 Hide M, Tanaka T, Yamamura Y, Koro O, Yamamoto S: IgE-mediated hypersensitivity against human sweat antigen in patients with atopic dermatitis. Acta Derm Venereol 2002;82:335–340.

9 Tanaka A, Tanaka T, Suzuki H, Ishii K, Kameyoshi Y, Hide M: Semi-purification of the immunoglobulin E-sweat antigen acting on mast cells and basophils in atopic dermatitis. Exp Dermatol 2006;15:283–290.
10 Shindo H, Ishii K, Yanase Y, Suzuki H, Hide M: Histamine release-neutralization assay for sera of patients with atopic dermatitis and/or cholinergic urticaria is useful to screen type I hypersensitivity against sweat antigens. Arch Dermatol Res 2012;304:647–654.
11 Sato K, Kang WH, Saga K, Sato KT: Biology of sweat glands and their disorders. I. Normal sweat gland function. J Am Acad Dermatol 1989;20:537–563.
12 Dai X, Okazaki H, Hanakawa Y, Murakami M, Tohyama M, Shirakata Y, Sayama K: Eccrine sweat contains IL-1α, IL-1β and IL-31 and activates epidermal keratinocytes as a danger signal. PLoS One 2013;8:e67666.
13 Yamaguchi H, Kabashima-Kubo R, Bito T, Sakabe J, Shimauchi T, Ito T, Hirakawa S, Hirasawa N, Ogasawara K, Tokura Y: High frequencies of positive nickel/cobalt patch tests and high sweat nickel concentration in patients with intrinsic atopic dermatitis. J Dermatol Sci 2013; 72:240–245.
14 Yamaguchi H, Hirasawa N, Asakawa S, Okita K, Tokura Y: Intrinsic atopic dermatitis shows high serum nickel concentration. Allergol Int 2015;64:282–284.
15 Valenta R, Maurer D, Steiner R, Seiberler S, Sperr WR, Valent P, Spitzauer S, Kapiotis S, Smolen J, Stingl G: Immunoglobulin E response to human proteins in atopic patients. J Invest Dermatol 1996;107:203–208.
16 Cipriani F, Ricci G, Leoni MC, Capra L, Baviera G, Longo G, Maiello N, Galli E: Autoimmunity in atopic dermatitis: biomarker or simply epiphenomenon? J Dermatol 2014;41:569–576.
17 Tang TS, Bieber T, Williams HC: Does 'autoreactivity' play a role in atopic dermatitis? J Allergy Clin Immunol 2012; 129:1209–1215.e2.
18 Vilhelmsson M, Johansson C, Jacobsson-Ekman G, Crameri R, Zargari A, Scheynius A: The *Malassezia sympodialis* allergen Mala s 11 induces human dendritic cell maturation, in contrast to its human homologue manganese superoxide dismutase. Int Arch Allergy Immunol 2007;143:155–162.
19 Balaji H, Heratizadeh A, Wichmann K, Niebuhr M, Crameri R, Scheynius A, Werfel T: *Malassezia sympodialis* thioredoxin-specific T cells are highly cross-reactive to human thioredoxin in atopic dermatitis. J Allergy Clin Immunol 2011;128:92–99.e4.
20 Lucae S, Schmid-Grendelmeier P, Wüthrich B, Kraft D, Valenta R, Linhart B: IgE responses to exogenous and endogenous allergens in atopic dermatitis patients under long-term systemic cyclosporine A treatment. Allergy 2016;71: 115–118.
21 Hiragun T, Ishii K, Hiragun M, Suzuki H, Kan T, Mihara S, Yanase Y, Bartels J, Schröder JM, Hide M: Fungal protein MGL_1304 in sweat is an allergen for atopic dermatitis patients. J Allergy Clin Immunol 2013;132:608–615.e4.
22 Hiragun M, Hiragun T, Ishii K, Suzuki H, Tanaka A, Yanase Y, Mihara S, Haruta Y, Kohno N, Hide M: Elevated serum IgE against MGL_1304 in patients with atopic dermatitis and cholinergic urticaria. Allergol Int 2014;63:83–93.
23 Ishii K, Hiragun M, Hiragun T, Kan T, Kawaguchi T, Yanase Y, Tanaka A, Takahagi S, Hide M: A human monoclonal IgE antibody that binds to MGL_1304, a major allergen in human sweat, without activation of mast cells and basophils. Biochem Biophys Res Commun 2015;468:99–104.
24 Kan T, Hiragun T, Ishii K, Hiragun M, Yanase Y, Tanaka A, Hide M: Evaluation of recombinant MGL_1304 produced by *Pichia pastoris* for clinical application to sweat allergy. Allergol Int 2015;64: 266–271.
25 Kameyoshi Y, Tanaka T, Mochizuki M, Koro O, Mihara S, Hiragun T, Tanaka M, Hide M: Taking showers at school is beneficial for children with severer atopic dermatitis (in Japanese). Arerugi 2008;57:130–137.
26 Mochizuki H, Muramatsu R, Tadaki H, Mizuno T, Arakawa H, Morikawa A: Effects of skin care with shower therapy on children with atopic dermatitis in elementary schools. Pediatr Dermatol 2009;26:223–225.
27 Chung SY, Reed S: Removing peanut allergens by tannic acid. Food Chem 2012;134:1468–1473.
28 Woodfolk JA, Hayden ML, Couture N, Platts-Mills TA: Chemical treatment of carpets to reduce allergen: comparison of the effects of tannic acid and other treatments on proteins derived from dust mites and cats. J Allergy Clin Immunol 1995;96:325–333.
29 Shindo H, Takahagi S, Mihara S, Tanaka T, Ishii K, Hide M, Suzuki S, Kanatani H, Yano S: Efficacy of sweat-antigen-inactivating skin care products on itching of patients with atopic dermatitis (in Japanese). Arerugi 2011;60:33–42.
30 Karuppagounder V, Arumugam S, Thandavarayan RA, Pitchaimani V, Sreedhar R, Afrin R, Harima M, Suzuki H, Nomoto M, Miyashita S, Suzuki K, Nakamura M, Ueno K, Watanabe K: Tannic acid modulates NFκB signaling pathway and skin inflammation in NC/Nga mice through PPARγ expression. Cytokine 2015;76:206–213.
31 Kozaru T, Fukunaga A, Taguchi K, Ogura K, Nagano T, Oka M, Horikawa T, Nishigori C: Rapid desensitization with autologous sweat in cholinergic urticaria. Allergol Int 2011;60:277–281.
32 Tanaka T, Ishii K, Suzuki H, Kameyoshi Y, Hide M: Cholinergic urticaria successfully treated by immunotherapy with partially purified sweat antigen (in Japanese). Arerugi 2007;56:54–57.

Michihiro Hide
Department of Dermatology, Integrated Health Sciences
Institute of Biomedical and Health Sciences, Hiroshima University
1-2-3 Kasumi, Minami-ku
Hiroshima 734-8551 (Japan)
E-Mail ed1h-w1de-road@hiroshima-u.ac.jp

Yokozeki H, Murota H, Katayama I (eds): Perspiration Research.
Curr Probl Dermatol. Basel, Karger, 2016, vol 51, pp 109–119 (DOI: 10.1159/000447370)

Perspiration Functions in Different Ethnic, Age, and Sex Populations: Modification of Sudomotor Function

Jeong Beom Lee[a] · Jeong Ho Kim[a] · Hiroyuki Murota[b]

[a]Department of Physiology, College of Medicine, Soonchunhyang University, Cheonan, Republic of Korea; [b]Department of Dermatology, Course of Integrated Medicine, Graduate School of Medicine, Osaka University, Osaka, Japan

Abstract

The sudomotor mechanism, wich contributes to tolerating thermal environments, is affected by not only the body temperature, but also sex, ethnicity, exercise training, region, season, and heat adaptation. Aging attenuates the sudomotor function by the decreased peripheral sensitivity to acetylcholine and demyelination of innervating nerves. Women show less sudomotor activity than men. Heat adaptation with sudomotor modification is induced by repetitive physical and/or thermal training. Short-term heat acclimation increases sweat gland activity. Long-term heat acclimation results in a reduction in the sweating response to stimuli. Residents of tropical areas sweat less and more slowly than residents of temperate areas. Short-term heat acclimation enhances the sweating response. Long-term heat acclimation, from seasonal change or migration, diminishes the sweating response. Also, deacclimation can be induced by migration from a tropical area to a temperate area. Body composition, especially brown adipose tissue, and weight affect thermal responses. Further studies should investigate BAT and endocrinal pyrogens as additional factors.

Humans can tolerate a wide range of thermal environments, but physiological function is dependent upon the maintenance of thermal homeostasis. When exposed to hyperthermic conditions, via environmental factors and/or increased metabolism, heat dissipation becomes vital for survival. In humans, the primary mechanism of heat dissipation is evaporative heat loss, secondary to sweat secretion from the eccrine glands. With a large surface area of hairless skin, sweating is an efficient evaporative cooling mechanism in humans. Evaporation of sweat is an important heat-loss process in the control of internal body temperature in a hot environment, in which the ambient temperature is higher than the skin temperature.

Central sudomotor mechanisms integrate inputs from the core and skin thermoreceptors, and produce signals to control the sweat glands [1–3]. Efferent sweat fibers originate in the preoptic area and anterior hypothalamus, and descend to the postganglionic sympathetic plexus (sudomotor neurons) through the ipsilateral brain stem and medulla [4]. The sweat glands generate a sweat response according to the central sudomotor nerve activity [1, 5–9]. In addition, peripheral conditions (local skin temperature and blood flow) can modulate the sweating response [10].

The autonomic nervous system regulates sudomotor function. Sudomotor response can be tested using several tools, such as thermoregulatory sweat testing, the Quantitative Sudomotor Axon Reflex Test (QSART), silicone impressions, the sympathetic skin response, the acetylcholine (ACh) sweat-spot test, and quantitative direct and indirect axon reflex testing [11]. QSART evaluates the postganglionic sympathetic sudomotor axons by measuring the axon reflex-mediated (AXR) and directly activated (DIR) sweat response over time, following stimulation of sweat glands with 10% ACh [4, 12, 13]. QSART has been a routine postganglionic sudomotor function (HCFA 95923) clinical laboratory test of the Mayo Clinic since 1983. DIR is based upon the response of muscarinic receptors, whereas AXR represents the nicotinic receptor response [12, 13]. Forearm sweat glands have been widely used to approximate sweating activity of the whole body [14, 15]. According to Low et al. [16], QSART provides close to maximal sweat gland stimulation. A large number of previous reports using QSART on the forearm have potentially demonstrated overall (whole body) sudomotor sensitivity.

Neural control of sweating, primarily regulated by the integration of internal and skin temperatures, is paramount for temperature regulation; however, a variety of other thermal and non-thermal factors also modify the sweating response. In this study we mainly focus on age, sex, ethnicity, exercise training, region, season, and heat adaptation.

Age and Sex

Numerous studies have used specific techniques to show that age and/or sex affect sudomotor function [1, 17–29]. Researchers have used ACh and/or methylcholine for sweating, and recruited specifically women or men, or subjects of both sexes, across various age groups. The results from such previous studies show that the attenuation of sudomotor function occurs with increased aging in both men and women. There is a progressive increase in onset time and a decrease in sweat rates, density of activated sweat glands (ASGs), and sweat output per gland (SGO), with increasing age in both sexes (fig. 1). A variation in sweat function between the sexes has been reported, but is not consistent in all age groups. Larose et al. [30] recently demonstrated, in a large sample of men between the ages of 20 and 70 years, that the capacity to dissipate heat was compromised as early as the age of 40 years, and declined progressively thereafter. Meanwhile, a slightly different approach is needed in the case of children. Araki et al. [31] and Shibasaki et al. [32] suggested that maturation is an important factor, as postadolescent subjects had a superior ability to activate sweat function compared with preadolescents during muscular exercise. Rees and Shuster [33] did not reveal a significant difference between sweat rates in prepubertal males and females.

There are several possible explanations for the apparent attenuation of sweating with ageing. Some researchers have suggested that the thermoregulation threshold (i.e. sweating threshold) is different between younger and older subjects, such that the threshold for the onset of sweating increases with ageing [22–24, 28]. The biological function of sweat glands stimulated by ACh be-

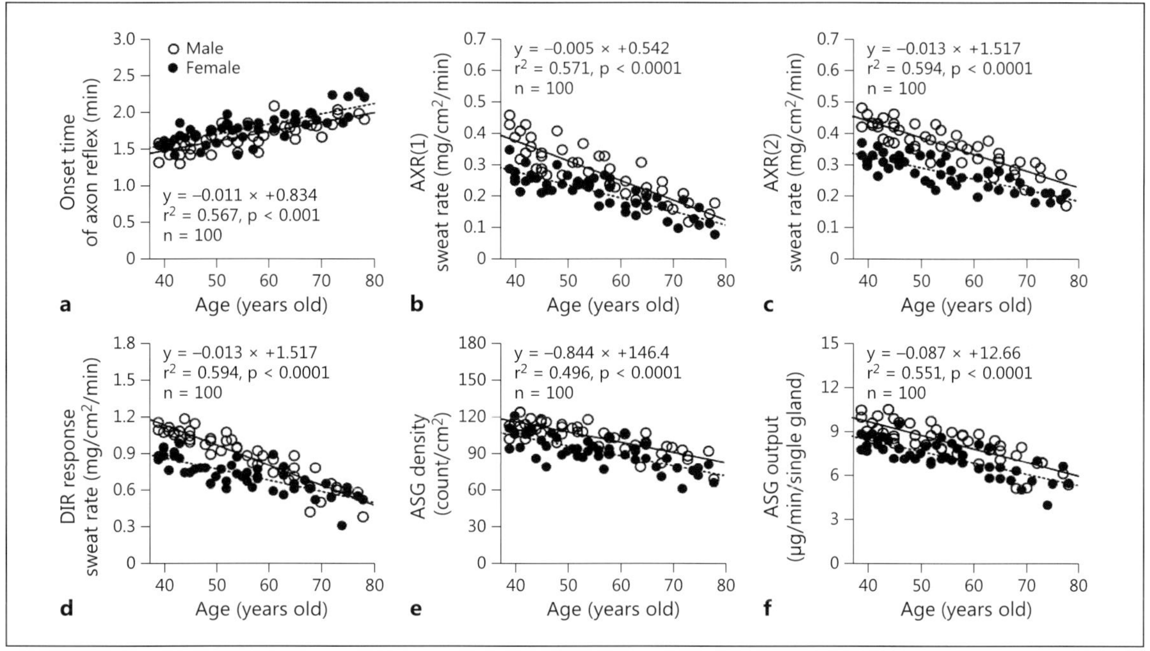

Fig. 1. A study [29] of the sudomotor function related to age and sex in healthy men (n = 52; ○) and healthy women (n = 48; ●) by QSART. **a** Sweating onset time of the AXR. **b** AXR(1) sweat rate, AXR(2) sweat rate. **c** DIR sweat rate. **d** ASG density. **e** Activated single SGO. AXR(1) = Sweating by axonal reflex, activating nicotinic receptor during iontophoresis; AXR(2) = local skin area where the sweating activity is induced by the nicotinic receptor: axonal reflex sweating after iontophoresis, for 5 min; DIR: direct responsive sweating induced by the muscarinic receptor after iontophoresis for 5 min. Sweating activities were compared after ACh iontophoresis. Correlation between onset time of the AXR sweating (**a**), AXR(1) sweating rate (**b**), AXR(2) sweating rate (**c**), DIR sweating rate (**d**), ASG density (**e**), ASG output (**f**), and age in male and female subjects.

comes lower with aging [28]. Inoue et al. [34] suggested that, as no significant change in the central sudomotor drive has been noted, the sluggish sweating response appears to be associated with age-related modifications in the periphery, involving reduced sweat gland sensitivity to cholinergic stimulation, or to sluggish vasodilatation. Low et al. [18] suggested that this change is caused by demyelination of the nerve fibers. Inoue et al. [35] demonstrated that SGO decreases gradually with age, due to progressive sweat gland atrophy. It has been postulated that the age-related impairments in sweating are due to differences in end-organ function, such as cholinergic sensitivity of the muscarinic receptors on the sweat glands [25, 26].

The nervous system, particularly postganglionic sympathetic nerve fibers that innervate sweat glands, degenerates with age. Namer et al. [36] showed that the physiological function of C-fibers declines with age and that mechanoresponsive C-fiber (classified afferent C-fiber) composition decreases to 58.5% in young subjects, compared with 39.6% in aged subjects, although the proportion of afferent and efferent fibers in young subjects is equal to those found in elderly subjects. Based on the data provided by Namer et al. [36], conduction velocity in aged subjects is slower than that of younger subjects, and the normalized time period is shorter in young subjects compared with that of aged subjects. Increases in sweating could be due to an increased density of ASGs, increased SGO, or a combination of both factors [37, 38]. Some researchers have demonstrated lower sweating rates in older subjects for a given pharmacological stimulus, attributable to a smaller output per activated gland but not density of ASG [25].

Aside from this, the anatomic alterations in cutaneous vessels (collapse, disorganization, and total disappearance in some cases) and diminished maximal skin blood flow capacities of older individuals [39], as well as augmented noradrenergic vasoconstriction [40], smaller increases in cardiac output, and redistribution of blood flow under heat stress [41], may also contribute to the limited thermal tolerance and depletion of sweating in older subjects.

Researchers generally agree that men sweat more than women [18, 42–44]. Women generally have less sweat gland secretory capacity than men, with lower maximal sweat rates, less of a response to local chemical stimulation, and a higher concentration of electrolytes in the sweat [42]. Low et al. [18] found from QSART data that men have approximately double the mean evoked sweat volume of women. Kihara et al. [45] reported that the density of ASGs does not differ between men and women, but the latter have a smaller evoked SGO. However, Lee et al. [29] observed significant differences in both density of ASGs and SGO.

Other variables, in addition to those mentioned above, that affect human perspiration require further investigation. Others include dynamic exercise or passive heat stress [46], dry or humid heat stress conditions [47], dose-dependent sweating response to the administration of ACh and methacholine [48, 49], hydration status, body surface area, etc., which also affect sudomotor function. Importantly, however, it is often difficult to separate the effects of each factor and concomitant influences. Researchers assume that there may be similar effects of an age-related decline in other physiological characteristics of subjects.

Heat Adaptation

Sudomotor activity is modified by repetitive physical and/or thermal training. Physical activities induce internal thermal loads and then raise the overall body temperature. Environmental heat or passive heating, such as hot water immersion, also increases body temperature and results in sweating. Repetitive physical activity or thermal load induces physiological heat adaptation in parallel with modified sudomotor activity. Sweating sensitivity depends on the extension of the period of acclimation [12]. The sweating reaction to short- and long-term acclimation differs.

Short-term heat acclimation occurs with an exposure time of 1–2 h a day, and can be complete within a few days and the 2nd week of exposure [50, 51]. Prior heat exposure, lasting several consecutive days, improves heat resistance [7, 52, 53] by increasing sweat output, lowering the heart rate, and slowing the rise in core temperature [3, 23, 53, 54]. Short-term heat acclimation reduces the initiation of sweating, and increases the amount of sweating [38]. Short-term heat acclimation increases sweat gland activity. In short-term heat acclimation trials, Taylor [55] and Sato et al. [52], observed increased sweat output, increased size of the eccrine sweat glands, and increased sensitivity of the sweat glands to methacholine stimulation. This increase in the volume of sweat allows the body to compensate for the increase in body temperature [56]. Reduced sweating initiation causes an acceleration of the peripheral sympathetic nervous system, which is considered advantageous in terms of energy dissipation for thermoregulation [4]. The enhanced sensitivity of the sweat glands appears to be due to increas-

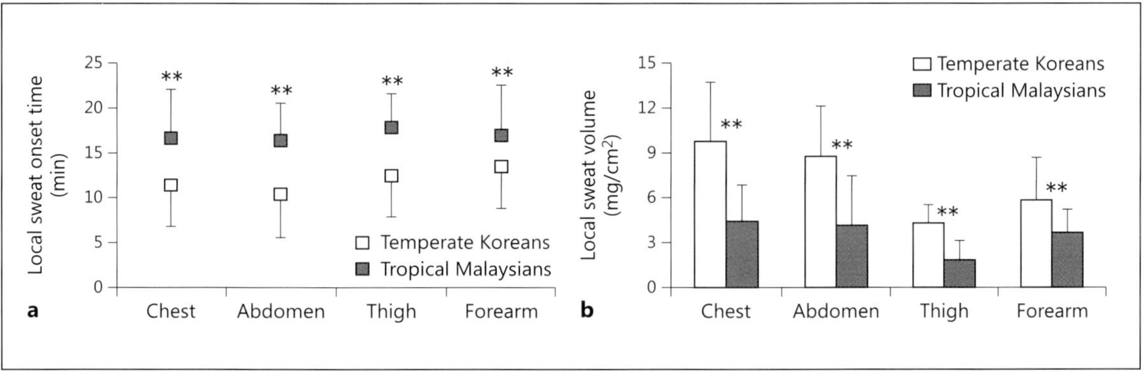

Fig. 2. Study of the CNS sudomotor sensitivity of tropical Malaysians and temperate Koreans (modification of Lee et al. [63]). A comparison of the local sweat onset time (**a**) and local sweat volume (**b**) on the chest, back, thigh, and forearm during heat load, induced via the immersion of the lower legs of temperate Korean (n = 13) and tropical Malaysian subjects (n = 10) in a hot water bath (43°C for 30 min). ** $p < 0.001$ between the groups (means ± SD).

es in direct and indirect sweating, active sweat gland density, and the output volume from individual sweat glands [4].

In contrast, heat acclimation over the longer term results in a reduction in the sweating response to stimuli [56, 57]. When long-term heat-acclimated subjects are compared to short-term heat-acclimated subjects following exposure to equal amounts of heat, the long-term heat-acclimated subjects sweat less [54, 58, 59]. When comparing tropical Africans to short-term heat-acclimated Japanese subjects, there is an increase in the threshold core temperature for sweating and a decreased ACh sensitivity in the Africans [60]. Lee et al. [56] also found that there is a lower volume of evaporative loss, lower sweat output, and a longer sweat onset time in Malaysian subjects. The suppressed sweating in tropical natives [12, 54, 58, 59] has the advantage of preserving body fluid by osmoregulation, so that individuals can better thermoregulate themselves [60].

Sensitivity to ACh may have been dulled following repeated stimulation of the sweat glands by heat-mediated release of endogenous ACh in hot and humid tropical climates [56]. The related finding that sensitivity of the sweat glands is diminished following repeated ACh administration supports this idea [6]. Both core and skin temperatures have a significant influence on the sweating response, not only as an input to the central regulatory mechanism, but also as a local control of sweat gland activity. Tropical subjects are able to maintain lower core and skin temperatures compared to temperate subjects [56, 58]. The size and number of ASGs can change upon heat exposure [53]. Lee et al. [56] demonstrated that lower sudomotor responses to ACh (suppressed ASG density and SGO) are indicative of dulled sympathetic nerve responsiveness to ACh. This physiological trait guarantees a more economical use of body fluids, thus ensuring more efficient protection against heat stress. In addition, long-term heat adaptation has provided evidence supporting a more effective convective heat transfer to the skin, and a more graded central control of sweating [61]. This points to adaptive adjustments of the central autonomic control in response to thermal adaptation, which should help to avoid excessive sweating and thereby contribute to improved body fluid homeostasis [61].

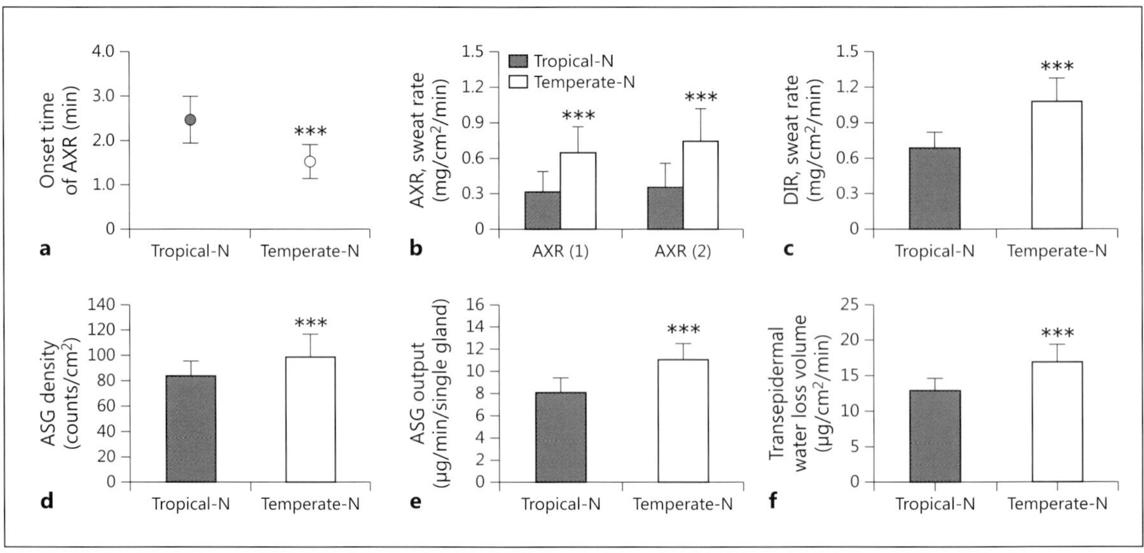

Fig. 3. Study on the peripheral nervous system sudomotor sensitivity of tropical Malaysians and temperate Koreans by QSART [57]. **a** Sweating onset time of the AXR. **b** AXR(1) sweat rate, AXR(2) sweat rate. **c** DIR sweat rate. **d** ASG density. **e** Activated single SGO. AXR(1) = Sweating by AXR, activating nicotinic receptor during iontophoresis, AXR(2) = local skin area where the sweating activity is induced by the nicotinic receptor: AXR sweating after iontophoresis, for 5 min; DIR = direct responsive sweating induced by muscarinic receptor after iontophoresis for 5 min. Sweating activities were compared after ACh iontophoresis. Compared with temperate Koreans, tropical Malaysians showed longer onset time of AXR (**a**), lower AXR(1), AXR(2), and DIR sweat rate (**b**, **c**), lower density of ASG (**d**), less SGO (**e**), and less evaporative water loss (**f**). Values are presented as means ± SD, statistically significant difference at *** $p < 0.001$. Temperate native (Temperate-N, n = 35) vs. tropical native (Tropical-N, n = 20) subjects.

Regional Differences of Sweating Activities

In the 1950s, Kuno [38] conducted real-time observations of sweating on the skin surface, and quantitated the density of ASGs in order to evaluate the differences between regions of difference environments. More recently, several studies have reported the regional differences of sweating activities between temperate Japanese and Africans [59], temperate Koreans and tropical Malaysians [56, 62], Thais [58], and Taiwanese and Filipinos [38]. Also, Africans have been shown to sweat less than Europeans during prolonged exercise in a hot and humid environment [59, 63].

Lee et al. [62] compared the sweating responses of temperate Koreans and tropical Malaysians to passive heating by leg immersion, with water at a temperature of 43°C in an air temperature of 25°C (fig. 2). In their study, the hygrometer capsule method was used; this method can measure the local sweat rate continuously by evaluating the humidity of the effluent gas from the capsule [62]. Comparing Koreans living in a temperate climate and Malaysians living in a tropical climate, the sweating onset time (chest, back, thigh, and forearm) of Malaysians was found to be significantly longer than for Koreans, and the local sweat rate (chest, back, thigh, and forearm) was lower in Malaysians than in Koreans [62].

These results [56] (fig. 3) suggest that suppressed thermal sweating in the tropical Malaysians is, at least in part, due to suppressed sweat gland sensitivity to ACh through both recruitment of ASGs and the SGO [56].

Also, in a study by Lee et al. [59] of Japanese and Africans using QSART, Africans presented slow sweating onset, lower sweating volume, lower density of ASGs, and lower SGOs [59].

Sweating Responses Due to Acclimation

Migration to regions of different climate and repeated thermal stimulation for some duration causes alteration of sweating response to heat stimulus. Nadel et al. [3] suggested a sweating model of a linear correlation between the central sweating drive and the sweating rate. The function of his sweating model can be transformed in two ways: change of slope and horizontal shift. These transformations result in a change in the potential sweating response for the given sweating drive. The two transformations correspond to the physical training and heat acclimation, respectively. Short-term heat acclimation occurs with an exposure of 1–2 h a day, and can be completed within a few days or by the second week of exposure [50, 51]. In the study by Lee et al. [4], an hour of leg immersion once a day for 10 days increases not only the evaporated quantity, but also ASG density and single SGO volume. These functional and anatomical changes are in agreement with the results of studies by Taylor [55] and Sato et al. [52], which showed increased sweat gland size and sensitivity to methacholine.

In long-term heat acclimation, thermal stimulation over a long period diminishes the sweating response to heat. Seasonal acclimation is one kind of long-term acclimation. Nakamura et al. [64] conducted a study on seasonal sweating variation of Japanese subjects living in Tokyo and Osaka, which have a temperate climate. In their study, air temperatue (T_a), skin temperature (T_{sk}), tympanic temperature (T_{ty}), and temperature change and sweating volume due to passive heating were measured across the studied year. In the time before summer, increased integrated sweating volume and decreased T_{ty} were shown in the short interval from June to August. Nakamura et al. [64] explained this rapid change using the sweating model of Nadel et al. [3]. Reinforced sweating due to a rise in T_a accelerated heat loss, causing T_{ty} and the onset threshold for T_{ty} to fall. During the time before winter, a gradual decrement of sweating from August to December was reported, and it is thought that reduced sweating, due to decreasing T_a, is alleviated by slightly increasing T_{ty} [64].

In a study by Lee et al. [65] regarding seasonal acclimation of young Korean adults, a coinciding tendency of response to passive heating was reported. The local sweating response of the subjects showed a shorter onset time and the sweating volume was greater at the summer seasonal acclimation (SA) state when compared to that of the winter SA. They were measured in July and January, respectively. In contrast, Lee et al. [65] reported that acclimation in a hot summer for 10 weeks led to decreased sweating volume and onset time in QSART. Measurements were taken twice, in July and September, when short- and long-term acclimation had taken place, respectively. As QSART can apply sufficient stimulus to elicit maximal sweating activity [16], it is inferred that peripheral sudomotor function is increased following summer acclimation.

The results of the studies by Nakamura et al. [64] and Lee [57] can be considered contradictory to each other; however, this can be explained by a different interpretation that integrates the time of measurement and the annual cycles of air temperature. In Korea and Japan, where the studies were completed, the highest temperatures are seen from July to September. In the study by Nakamura et al. [64], considering that heat acclimation needed a certain duration to be accomplished, the maximal sweating response in August can be understood to be a result of the temperature which is on the increase from June onwards, and this is the duration in which short-term acclimation is expected. From August to October, the sweating response was shown to decrease, and this also should not be considered to be as a result of the temperature at that time, but instead as a result of long-term acclimation due to the high temperature from July to September. In other words, although it is confirmed that the summer season shows a higher active sweating response than in winter, the time of the highest air temperature does not coincide with the time of the strongest sweating. The tendency of sweating does not coincide with T_a and T_{sk}, but increases in early summer, and falls later in the summer. This reasoning can explain the contradictions of the three aforementioned studies.

Seasonal variation can be impaired by lifestyle. In seasonal acclimation, basal metabolic rate alters with core temperature and sudomotor activity [65]. Sawka [51] highlighted a dwindling amplitude of seasonal changes in basal metabolic rate. The penetration of air conditioners or the changing of the dietary lifestyle could be an explanation of this recent impaired acclimation. A study by Bain and Jay [66] showed diminished acclimation due to behavioral adaptation. Measurements of core temperatures (esophageal, rectal, and tympanic), mean skin temperature, sweating, and skin blood flow before and after summer gave no statistically significant difference. Indoor activity with air conditioning comprised much of the physical activity records of the subjects involved.

Reduced sweating can be achieved by direct stimulus across a period of just several days, not only during long durations of seasonal change. Chen and Elizondo [6] administered ACh 4 times a day for 9 days, and the subjects' local sweating by passive heating was almost completely suppressed. This result implies that decreased thermal sweating can result from the desensitization of the nerve-gland interface derived from repetitive stimulation.

Acclimation by migration creates a dramatic alteration in sweating activity. Bae et al. [12] compared QSART of Japanese subjects living in temperate and tropical regions for at least 2 years. They found that the longer the tropical subjects lived in the tropical region, the more their sweating decreased and onset time increased. Also, in a study by Matsumoto et al. [58], subjects that migrated from cold to tropical regions showed substantial increases in sweat output initially, but this began to decrease several years later.

On the other hand, subjects that migrated from tropical or subtropical to temperate regions experienced declamation. Lee et al. [13] confirmed that Malaysians who lived in Japan for various durations (from 2 to 72 months) demonstrated this correlation between a short sweating onset time and large sweating volume with the duration of residence. In another study, the sweating response of migrants from Okinawa (subtropical) who lived for less than 3 years or longer than 10 years on the Japanese mainland (temperate) were compared [67]. The former had a lower sweating response on passive heating and higher thermal resistance than the latter. Saat et al. [68] reported that Malaysians who lived in Japan for more than 27 months showed a shorter sweating onset time on QSART than those who lived in Japan for less than 15 months. In addition, Wijayanto et al. [69] performed leg immersion to tropical natives that had lived in Japan for 4–47 months and found a coinciding correlation between sweating onset time and total body sweating rate with the duration of residence.

Individual and Racial Physical Factors Affecting Thermoregulation

Several individual factors affect human physiological responses to heat and cold, and subsequent adaptation. Body composition and weight were observed to affect the thermal responses [70]. As such, it is possible that weight and body fat during different seasons may be associated with seasonal changes in sweating responses. Brown adipose tissue (BAT) is found in high proportions in young men, but the metabolic action of BAT is reduced in overweight and obese subjects [71]. A previous study found both photoperiod and ambient temperature to have a strong impact on BAT expression and function [72]. Therefore, further studies are needed to elucidate the sweating responses involved in body composition depending on the season.

Regarding racial factors or genetic factors, Wijayanto et al. [69] stated that heat acclimation in tropical natives is a reflection of their physiological adjustment to environmental factors rather than the involvement of genetic factors, considering several results of acclimation of migrants. However, the effect of racial factors or genetic factors on thermal acclimation remains to be found.

Lee et al. [59] reported that, when comparing temperate Japanese and tropical Africans, longer sweating onset time and lower sweating volume, lower density of ASGs and lower SGO were seen in Africans. The results correspond with the results of our previous study, where we performed QSART on Koreans and Malaysians, as presented in figure 1a–e [56].

However, while African subjects [59] are in accordance with Allen's law [73], which says high temperature regions frequently have a slim body type with thin and long extremities, Malaysian subjects [56] have the typical Asian body type, which is similar to that of Koreans or Japanese. Therefore, further studies should investigate BAT and endocrinal pyrogens, rather than solely heat conductivity related with thickness of subcutaneous fat, body type, and body surface area, which are already known.

References

1 Taniguchi Y, et al: Contribution of central versus sweat gland mechanisms to the seasonal change of sweating function in young sedentary males and females. Int J Biometeorol 2011;55:203–212.

2 Henane R, Valatx JL: Thermoregulatory changes induced during heat acclimatization by controlled hypothermia in man. J Physiol 1973;230:255–271.

3 Nadel ER, Pandolf KB, Roberts M, et al: Mechanisms of thermal acclimation to exercise and heat. J Appl Physiol 1974; 37:515–520.

4 Lee JB, Kim TW, Shin YO, et al: Effect of the heat-exposure on peripheral sudomotor activity including the density of active sweat glands and single sweat gland output. Korean J Physiol Pharmacol 2010;14:273–278.

5 Collins KJ, Crockford GW, Weiner JS: The local training effect of secretory activity on the response of eccrine sweat glands. J Physiol 1966;184:203–214.

6 Chen WY, Elizondo RS: Peripheral modification of thermoregulatory function during heat acclimation. J Appl Physiol 1974;37:367–373.

7 Sato K, Sato F: Individual variations in structure and function of human eccrine sweat gland. Am J Physiol 1983; 245:R203–R208.

8 Buono MJ, McKenzie BK, Kasch FW: Effects of ageing and physical training on the peripheral sweat production of the human eccrine sweat gland. Age Ageing 1991;20:439–441.

9 Provitera V, et al: Evaluation of sudomotor function in diabetes using the dynamic sweat test. Neurol 2010;74: 50–56.

10 Wingo JE, et al: Skin blood flow and local temperature independently modify sweat rate during passive heat stress in humans. J Appl Physiol 2010;109:1301–1306.

11 Illigens BM, Gibbons CH: Sweat testing to evaluate autonomic function. Clin Auton Res 2009;19:79–87.

12 Bae JS, Lee JB, Matsumoto, et al: Prolonged residence of temperate natives in the tropics produces a suppression of sweating. Pflugers Arch 2006;453:67–72.

13 Lee JB, Bae JS, Lee MY, et al: The change in peripheral sweating mechanisms of the tropical Malaysian who stays in Japan. J Therm Biol 2004;29: 743–747.

14 Kondo N, Yanagimoto S, Aoki K, et al: Effect of activated sweat glands on the intensity-dependent sweating response to sustained static exercise in mildly heated humans. Jpn J Physiol 2002;52:229–233.

15 Ogawa T, Asayama M, Miyagawa T: Effects of sweat gland training by repeated local heating. Jpn J Physiol 1982;32:971–981.

16 Low PA, Opfer-Gehrking TL, Kihara M: In vivo studies on receptor pharmacology of the human eccrine sweat gland. Clin Auton Res 1992;2:29–34.

17 McGann KP, Marion GS, Camp L, et al: The influence of gender and race on mean body temperature in a population of healthy older adults. Arch Fam Med 1993;2:1265–1267.

18 Low PA, et al: Effect of age and gender on sudomotor and cardiovagal function and blood pressure response to tilt in normal subjects. Muscle Nerve 1997;20: 1561–1568.

19 Kaciuba-Uscilko H, Grucza R: Gender differences in thermoregulation. Curr Opin Clin Nutr Metab Care 2001;4:533–536.

20 Anderson RK, Kenney WL: Effect of age on heat-activated sweat gland density and flow during exercise in dry heat. J Appl Physiol 1987;63:1089–1094.

21 Dufour A, Candas V: Ageing and thermal responses during passive heat exposure: sweating and sensory aspects. Eur J Appl Physiol 2007;100:19–26.
22 Hellon RF, Lind AR: Observations on the activity of sweat glands with special reference to the influence of ageing. J Physiol 1956;133:132–144.
23 Wyndham CH: Effect of acclimatization on the sweat rate-rectal temperature relationship. J Appl Physiol 1967;22: 27–30.
24 Inbar O, Morris N, Epstein Y, et al: Comparison of thermoregulatory responses to exercise in dry heat among prepubertal boys, young adults and older males. Exp Physiol 2004;89:691–700.
25 Kenney WL, Fowler SR: Methylcholine-activated eccrine sweat gland density and output as a function of age. J Appl Physiol 1988;65:1082–1086.
26 Inoue Y, Havenith G, Kenney WL, et al: Exercise- and methylcholine-induced sweating responses in older and younger men: effect of heat acclimation and aerobic fitness. Int J Biometeorol 1999;42: 210–216.
27 Gagnon D, Crandall CG, Kenny GP: Sex differences in postsynaptic sweating and cutaneous vasodilation. J Appl Physiol 2013;114:394–401.
28 Foster KG, Ellis FP, Dore C, Exton-Smith AN, Weiner JS: Sweat responses in the aged. Age Ageing 1976;5:91–101.
29 Lee JB, Lee IH, Shin YO, et al: Age- and sex-related differences in sudomotor function evaluated by the Quantitative Sudomotor Axon Reflex Test (QSART) in healthy humans. Clin Exp Pharmacol Physiol 2014;41:392–399.
30 Larose J, Boulay P, Sigal RJ, et al: Age-related decrements in heat dissipation during physical activity occur as early as the age of 40. PLoS One 2013;8:e83148.
31 Araki T, Toda Y, Matsushita K, et al: Age differences in sweating during muscular exercise. J Phys Fitness Sports Med 1979;28:239–248.
32 Shibasaki M, Inoue Y, Kondo N, et al: Thermoregulatory responses of prepubertal boys and young men during moderate exercise. Eur J Appl Physiol Occup Physiol 1997;75:212–218.
33 Rees J, Shuster S: Pubertal induction of sweat gland activity. Clin Sci 1981;60: 689–692.
34 Inoue Y, Shibasaki M, Ueda H, et al: Mechanisms underlying the age-related decrement in the human sweating response. Eur J Appl Physiol Occup Physiol 1999;79:121–126.
35 Inoue Y, Kuwahara T, Araki T: Maturation- and aging-related changes in heat loss effector function. J Physiol Anthropol Appl Human Sci 2004;23:289–294.
36 Namer B, et al: Microneurographic assessment of C-fibre function in aged healthy subjects. J Physiol 2009;587: 419–428.
37 Kondo N, et al: Regional differences in the effect of exercise intensity on thermoregulatory sweating and cutaneous vasodilation. Acta Physiol Scand 1998; 164:71–78.
38 Kuno Y: Human Perspiration. Springfield, Charles C. Thomas, 1956.
39 Minson CT, Holowatz LA, Wong BJ, et al: Decreased nitric oxide- and axon reflex-mediated cutaneous vasodilation with age during local heating. J Appl Physiol (1985) 2002;93:1644–1649.
40 Kenney WL, et al: Decreased active vasodilator sensitivity in aged skin. Am J Physiol 1997;272:H1609–H1614.
41 Minson CT, Wladkowski SL, Cardell AF, et al: Age alters the cardiovascular response to direct passive heating. J Appl Physiol (1985) 1998;84:1323–1332.
42 Morimoto T, Slabochova Z, Naman RK, et al: Sex differences in physiological reactions to thermal stress. J Appl Physiol 1967;22:526–532.
43 Low PA, Caskey PE, Tuck RR, et al: Quantitative sudomotor axon reflex test in normal and neuropathic subjects. Ann Neurol 1983;14:573–580.
44 Low PA, Opfer-Gehrking TL, Proper CJ, et al: The effect of aging on cardiac autonomic and postganglionic sudomotor function. Muscle Nerve 1990;13:152–157.
45 Kihara M, Opfer-GehrkingTL, Low PA: Comparison of directly stimulated with axon-reflex-mediated sudomotor responses in human subjects and in patients with diabetes. Muscle Nerve 1993; 16:655–660.
46 Kondo N, et al: Function of human eccrine sweat glands during dynamic exercise and passive heat stress. J Appl Physiol (1985) 2001;90:1877–1881.
47 Larose J, et al: Age-related differences in heat loss capacity occur under both dry and humid heat stress conditions. J Appl Physiol (1985) 2014;117:69–79.
48 Smith CJ, Alexander LM, Kenney WL, et al: Age-related decrements in regional sweating and skin blood flow. Am J Physiol Regul Integr Comp Physiol 2013;305:R877–R885.
49 Stapleton JM, Fujii N, McGinn R et al: Age-related differences in postsynaptic increases in sweating and skin blood flow postexercise. Physiol Rep 2014; 2:e12078.
50 Pandolf KB: Time course of heat acclimation and its decay. Int J Sports Med 1998;19(suppl 2):S157–S160.
51 Sawka MN: Thermoregulatory responses to acute exercise heat stress and acclimation; in Fregly MJ, Blatteis CM (eds): Handbook of Physiology, Section 4. Environmental Physiology. New York, Oxford University Press, 1996.
52 Sato F, Owen M, Matthes R, Sato K, et al: Functional and morphological changes in the eccrine sweat gland with heat acclimation. J Appl Physiol (1985) 1990; 69:232–236.
53 Nielsen B: Heat acclimation – mechanisms of adaptation to exercise in the heat. Int J Sports Med 1998;19(suppl 2):S154–S156.
54 Ogawa T, Sugenoya J: Pulsatile sweating and sympathetic sudomotor activity. Jpn J Physiol 1993;43:275–289.
55 Taylor NA: Eccrine sweat glands. Adaptations to physical training and heat acclimation. Sports Med 1986;3:387–397.
56 Lee JB, Bae JS, Matsumoto T, et al: Tropical Malaysians and temperate Koreans exhibit significant differences in sweating sensitivity in response to iontophoretically administered acetylcholine. Int J Biometeorol 2009;53:149–157.
57 Lee JB: Heat acclimatization in hot summer for ten weeks suppress the sensitivity of sweating in response to iontophoretically-administered acetylcholine. Kor J Physiol Pharmacol 2008;12:349–355.
58 Matsumoto T, Yamauchi M, Tsuchiya K, et al: Study on mechanisms of heat acclimatization due to thermal sweating-comparison of heat tolerance between Japanese and Thai subjects. Trop Med 1993;35:23–34.

59 Lee JB, Othman T, Kosaka M, et al: Suppression of the sweat gland sensitivity to acetylcholine applied iontophoretically in tropical Africans compared to temperate Japanese. Trop Med 1997;39: 111–121.
60 Sawka MN, Coyle EF: Influence of body water and blood volume on thermoregulation and exercise performance in the heat. Exerc Sport Sci Rev 1999;27:167–218.
61 Yamauchi M, Matsumoto T, Ohwatari N, et al: Sweating economy by graded control in well-trained athletes. Pflugers Arch 1997;433:675–678.
62 Lee JB, Shin YO, Kang JC, et al: Long-term tropical residency diminishes central sudomotor sensitivities in male subjects. Korean J Physiol Pharmacol 2007; 11:233–237.
63 Wyndham CH, et al: Heat reactions of Caucasians in temperate, in hot, dry, and in hot, humid climates. J Appl Physiol 1964;19:607–612.
64 Nakamura Y, Okamura K: Seasonal variation of sweating responses under identical heat stress. Appl Human Sci 1998; 17:167–172.
65 Lee JB, Kim TW, Min YK, et al: Seasonal acclimatization in summer versus winter to changes in the sweating response during passive heating in Korean young adult men. Korean J Physiol Pharmacol 2015;19:9–14.
66 Bain AR, Jay O: Does summer in a humid continental climate elicit an acclimatization of human thermoregulatory responses? Eur J Appl Physiol 2011;111: 1197–1205.
67 Hori S, et al: Effect of long term residence in the temperate zone on the physique and sweating reaction of subtropical natives. Int J Biometeorol 1979;23: 255–261.
68 Saat M, Lee JB, Matsumoto T, et al: Relationship between the duration of stay in Japan of Malaysian subjects and the suppression of sweat gland sensitivity by Iontophoretically applied acetylcholine. Acta Med Nagasaki 1999;44:49–53.
69 Wijayanto T, Toramoto S, Wakabayashi H, et al: Effects of duration of stay in temperate area on thermoregulatory responses to passive heat exposure in tropical south-east Asian males residing in Japan. J Physiol Anthropol 2012;31: 25.
70 Sawka MN, Montain SJ, Latzka WA: Hydration effects on thermoregulation and performance in the heat. Comp Biochem Physiol A Mol Integr Physiol 2001;128:679–690.
71 Bittel JH: Heat debt as an index for cold adaptation in men. J Appl Physiol (1985) 1987;62:1627–1634.
72 van Marken Lichtenbelt WD, et al: Cold-activated brown adipose tissue in healthy men. N Engl J Med 2009;360: 1500–1508.
73 Persichetti A, Sciuto R, Rea S, et al: Prevalence, mass, and glucose-uptake activity of 18F-FDG-detected brown adipose tissue in humans living in a temperate zone of Italy. PLoS One 2013; 8:e63391.

Prof. Jeong-Beom Lee, MD, PhD
Department of Physiology
College of Medicine
Soonchunhyang University
366-1 Ssang Yong-dong
Cheonan 331-946 (Republic of Korea)
E-Mail leejb@sch.ac.kr

Author Index

Subject Index